PRAISE FOR
ROOM AT THE TABLE

Renee's book is a game-changing requisite toolkit for modern leadership. It urges leaders to aim at transforming laws and policies and the very foundations of our thoughts, mindsets, and hearts. This book is a clarion call for those willing to take on the toughest of tasks, championing for equality while navigating the complexities of leadership. Its unique narrative reinforces the notion that leading is not merely about imposing rules, but about inspiring a deep-seated shift in our beliefs and attitudes. The author compellingly challenges leaders to engage in "heart work"—a sincere commitment toward fostering understanding, compassion, and justice in society. *Room at the Table* is more than a manual—it is a manifesto for those daring enough to spark enduring change and a testament to the power of courageous leadership. This is an essential read for anyone seeking to make an impact, inspire change, and lead with authenticity and bravery.

—ERIC D. THOMAS, PHD

#1 motivational speaker,
New York Times best-selling author of You Owe You

In this compelling narrative Dr. Renee Branch Canady shares the profound wisdom gained from her lived experiences as a Black woman finding her voice, investing her talents, and navigating personal and professional challenges as she rises to lead large academic nursing and public health organizations. Filled with compelling data, thought-provoking ideas, and introspective storytelling, *Room at the Table* is an essential and inspiring read for those who seek to lead our society toward equity, justice, and health.

—LISA A. COOPER, MD, MPH
*2007 MacArthur Fellow, Director, Johns Hopkins Center for Health Equity,
author of* Why Are Health Disparities Everyone's Problem?

Room at the Table is a memoir of identity, purpose, and justice that delves into Dr. Renee Canady's personal and professional journey as a Black woman and health equity leader. She offers a candid account of her experiences and the insights she has gained along the way. From growing up in a military family to finding her passion in public health and advocating for social justice, her story is both relatable and inspiring. By weaving together personal anecdotes, historical context, and thought-provoking questions, this book challenges readers to examine their own lives and strive for a more equitable and inclusive society.

—DEBRA FURR-HOLDEN, PHD
Dean, New York University School of Global Public Health

In *Room at the Table* Dr. Renee Canady gives the reader the unique opportunity to challenge both the head and the heart in order to authentically promote and practice health equity. I would recommend this book for any leader who wishes to dismantle and destroy the mental and physical health disparities that painfully still exist for diverse community members. By the end of this important work, you too will be convinced that there is indeed room at the table for all.

— GLORIA MORROW, PHD
Clinical Psychologist, Director of Behavioral Health,
Unicare Community Health Center, Inc., DEIB Consultant and Author

ROOM AT THE TABLE

DR. RENÉE BRANCH CANADY

ROOM AT THE TABLE

A LEADER'S GUIDE TO ADVANCING HEALTH EQUITY AND JUSTICE

Advantage | Books

Published by Advantage Books, Charleston, South Carolina.
An imprint of Advantage Media.

ADVANTAGE is a registered trademark, and the Advantage colophon is a trademark of Advantage Media Group, Inc.

Printed in the United States of America.

10 9 8 7 6 5 4 3 2 1

ISBN: 978-1-64225-657-4 (Paperback)
ISBN: 978-1-64225-656-7 (eBook)

Library of Congress Control Number: 2023911378

Cover design by Josh Frederick.
Layout design by Matthew Morse.

This publication is designed to provide accurate and authoritative information in regard to the subject matter covered. It is sold with the understanding that the publisher is not engaged in rendering legal, accounting, or other professional services. If legal advice or other expert assistance is required, the services of a competent professional person should be sought.

Advantage Books is an imprint of Advantage Media Group. Advantage Media helps busy entrepreneurs, CEOs, and leaders write and publish a book to grow their business and become the authority in their field. Advantage authors comprise an exclusive community of industry professionals, idea-makers, and thought leaders. For more information go to **advantagemedia.com**.

For Howard, whose short life continues to shape mine.
For Bernice, whose shortened life gave foundation to mine.
For Mamie, whose long life guided mine.

To Marcus, Alexander, and Wesley.
Your lives matter and make a difference every day.
I love you each beyond measure and end.

CONTENTS

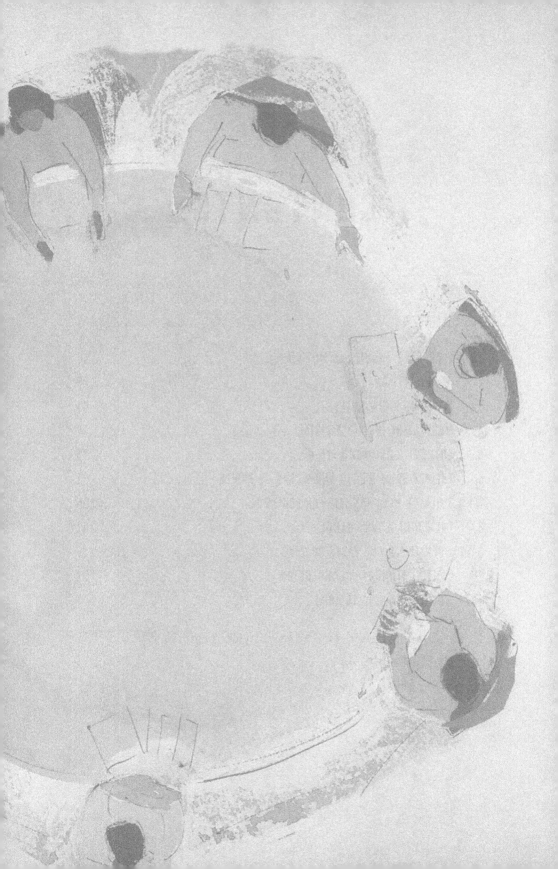

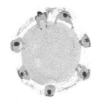

INTRODUCTION

Honesty and openness is always the foundation
of insightful dialogue.

—BELL HOOKS

So I finally decided to capture my thoughts and learnings in a book. Colleagues and friends have repeatedly urged me to do so, and at last, I have acquiesced. But a book about what and to whom? I began reflecting on my own identities and responsibilities to help gain clarity on this foundational decision. I am a mother, sister, daughter, administrator, public health professional, follower of Jesus Christ, minister of the gospel, and singer. Fundamentally, I'm an equity leader, and I wish to inspire those who choose this path while giving voice to all the other roles they play in life. Yes, this book is for the secular and the spiritual space, as well as academic and professional spaces. What you're reading isn't as important as what you think about what you're reading, what you feel about what you're reading, and what you will consequently do.

Because I am a Black woman and health equity leader, *Room at the Table* is informed by my lived experiences as an author and storyteller, as well as my relationship with knowledge and ways of knowing.

It is presented in a classic textbook manner because of the patterns represented. It is nonfiction, as it highlights and analyzes realities, and it is also fiction in that it presents an aspirational, perhaps unattainable utopia that we must somehow pursue. As you can already tell, this isn't purely an instructional manual—there are plenty of books that are technical and research driven. *Room at the Table* is intentionally an equity leadership guide that uses narrative and storytelling to bring to life the experiences that I've had as a leader. It is also a model to bring to life *your* stories.

On that note, let's begin with my beginnings.

I grew up in a military family. When I was seven, my father received new orders from the US Air Force. We were moving to Arizona. Traveling was always an exciting time for me! When we drove there, I just assumed our meticulous method of travel was how everyone moved or took a road trip—make a bunch of sandwiches, pack up other snacks for the car, and keep driving until you find a space to pull over for the night. You know, so Dad can sleep. Wasn't this how all people traveled? *No.*

I didn't realize that we were going through areas that were not necessarily safe spaces for a Black family. My parents didn't know whether or not we'd encounter a community that would welcome our presence at dine-in restaurants. In terms of the law, we could *legally* go in, but I imagine my parents asking themselves, "Do we want to expose our kids to something like that?" The stares, the questions, the backlash. Ah, it was age and experience that brought this reflective realization …

Another pivotal event for me growing up involved my "best friend in the world." She had a birthday slumber party, and everyone was invited except for her best friend—me. That's when my mom and I had the talk. The *race* talk. I believed my parents when they told me how wonderful I was. They even gave me the nickname "Princess." My reaction then was, *How awful for my best friend and her guests!* I would have been a lot of fun at that party. And again, a reflective realization ...

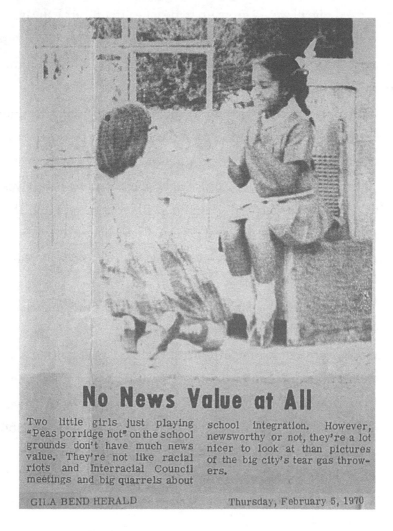

No News Value at All

Two little girls just playing "Peas porridge hot" on the school grounds don't have much news value. They're not like racial riots and Interracial Council meetings and big quarrels about school integration. However, newsworthy or not, they're a lot nicer to look at than pictures of the big city's tear gas throwers.

GILA BEND HERALD   Thursday, February 5, 1970

This photo was published in a small-town Arizona newspaper, the *Gila Bend Herald*, in 1970 entitled "No News Value at All."

"Two little girls just playing Peas Porridge Hot on the school grounds don't have much news value. They're not like racial riots and interracial council meetings, and big quarrels about school integration. However newsworthy or not, they're a lot nicer to look at than pictures of the big city's tear gas throwers."

Significant. Who would've thought that same little Black girl with the crooked pigtail would grow up to be a health officer? I always had self-confidence. I had assumed I'd attend the birthday party, but I didn't get the invitation. This moment shaped me, and I'll ask many times, What moments have shaped *you*?

From a young age, I could already see how deeply wounded people are on both sides of the color line. How many other gatherings were robbed of richness because people are locked in these closed paradigms, missing the opportunity to be their absolute best selves—closing off to those who had something different to give and share? As an extroverted child who loved friends—which now translates into my adult drive for relationships—I knew I wanted to "fix" these issues that damaged relationships.

When I earned my degree in public health at the University of North Carolina, it was almost as an afterthought. It was my second bachelor's degree and something to do while I pursued my dream of moving on to medical school. My mother was a public health nurse and couldn't help but ask, "Are you sure you want to go to medical school? Medicine is a very demanding field. Think about all the things you like to do, like community theater, singing, and traveling!" I already had a bachelor's in zoology and sang in the UNC Black Student Movement Gospel Choir, so my mom had a point. I had many interests.

I affirmed that I wanted to attend medical school and be in charge! My mom was an accomplished nurse leader, but I wanted to be the *doctor*. I sadly lost my mother—my friend and confidant—to breast cancer as my medical educational journey moved forward. I like to joke that my mom got in front of God and requested, "Get this hardheaded daughter of mine into nursing." While I'm not a nurse or physician today, I've spent my career partnering with nurses—working for them, supervising them, and then advocating and cheering for more people to go into nursing. My mother's legacy and influence live on as I continue to steep myself in her passion for public health.

The skeleton in my closet is that I spent two years in medical school figuring out I didn't want to be a physician after all. That was a very expensive way to enact career planning! In truth, I was miserable, but I had the serendipitous moment of failing a pivotal class and figured I needed to listen to the signs. I had to move on, and a move to Lansing, Michigan, found me gaining employment in my first public health job. It was the mideighties, and I found myself in the early years of our fight against the AIDS/HIV epidemic.

At the time, it was called HTLV-III, and we had no clear idea what was happening. Public narrative managed to distinguish "innocent victims" (children with hemophilia or those who'd received "tainted" blood transfusions) from others who were labeled and presumed guilty ("drug addicts" and "homosexuals"). Our collective propensity for alienating and *othering* was fully displayed. My commitment to health equity and social justice began after seeing the horrible physical and mental health consequences of people being condemned and treated poorly simply because of who they are. I had to ask myself, *How can I help people see who others* are *rather than what they've done or experienced?* How could we not see their humanity—wonderful people who had gotten sick? Why were others dehumanizing them?

other:

gerund or present participle: othering.

To view or treat (a person or group of people) as intrinsically different from and alien to oneself.

After this period, my career focus shifted to adolescent health and teen pregnancy. I was proud to lead a comprehensive adolescent program that included healthcare, education, and support for young people with unique needs, including runaways and teen moms. Next, I was recruited back into HIV prevention in partnership with the state's Department of Corrections and the Department of Community Health. After this, the College of Nursing at Michigan State University (MSU) lured me in (another subtle heavenly wink from my mom!). I led a program focused on recruiting underrepresented students into the profession, ushering men and students of color into the field.

While working at MSU, I decided it was the perfect opportunity to deal with that skeleton in my closet—the unfinished doctoral degree. When talking with a friend, I mentioned that I never wanted to practice medicine. I didn't want to be the "Stick out your tongue and say *ahh*" doctor. I wanted to be an advocate who thought about what happens to people when they *get* sick—the context of their lives and how their families are affected. How does a family take the difficult journey together? What is their experience like versus the neighbors' experiences? How might experiences vary across racial groups, and do those diverse experiences affect health outcomes?

With a *matter-of-fact* undertone, my friend asked, "Why didn't you just study medical sociology?" I thought I could either pretend like I knew what that was or do the research and learn. That's precisely what I did. As it turned out, MSU had an excellent program. I experienced outstanding mentorship, focusing my work on researching infant mortality and the pregnancy outcomes of Black women—analyzing the pregnancy experience differences between Black and white women. My mentor advised me to focus on something fueled by passion and purpose—something that, when you're up at 2:00 a.m. writing that dissertation all by yourself, will keep you driving.

I have a history of alcoholism in my family, so I could have chosen that research topic. I've experienced and survived divorce and could have researched that subject. My mother's premature death from breast cancer had a significant impact on our family—certainly another worthy topic to investigate. But I knew the memory of my son, Mark Howard, would keep me driving and pushing. Indeed, his memory did and still does.

I have always been a well-resourced, well-supported Black woman (recognizing that the finances ebbed and flowed over my journey). My mother, *the nurse*, taught me an appreciation for my body and the changes that would happen as a woman. And so it seemed as though I knew precisely when I conceived my son, Howard. Similarly, it would seem that mother wit was my grandmother's skill—she could see what I could not. Grandtie, as we called her, had been a nurse's aide. People just adored her. She was one of those magnetic, witty personalities that everyone wanted to be around.

During my pregnancy, my husband was campaigning for city council. We were out and about, and everyone saw us as this model young couple—the politician and his pregnant wife—just the perfect picture! However, my grandmother kept commenting, "I don't like the way the back of your legs look." I'd ask her what she was talking about. "Well, they just look a little … a little bit *puffy*." I thought my calves were fine, but she persisted. "Well, how about your feet?"

Sure, they were swollen—I was pregnant—and in my mind they weren't *that* swollen. I look back on this experience and ask myself, *What was my grandmother seeing?* She told me to put my feet up, rub my legs with liniment—do this and do that. I did it all because I was trying to indulge my grandmother while assuming that I was fine. Preeclampsia was the condition that led to my son's early delivery. It was one of those silent and sudden things, as hypertension can be. The condition is harmful to the mother as well as the child. He was born in May and thrived until cold and flu season arrived. In December, he caught respiratory syncytial virus—RSV. That was too much for his young vulnerable lungs to fight off. I am grateful for the six months of memories with my son.

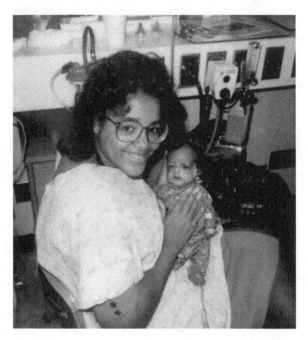

with Mark Howard II (May 1989–December 1989)

My son died in 1989 at Sparrow Hospital in Ingham County. As I'm composing this introduction, it's my son's birthday. He would have been thirty-three years old today. As it turns out, Black women have the highest age-adjusted prevalence of preeclampsia. It is my hope that this book summons equity leaders to ask why.

My own desire to know why pushed me ahead. I stood simultaneously as a motherless child and a childless mother. No one wants to be a member of the "I lost a child" club … I didn't want this membership card, but the card opened up so many opportunities for me to be a blessing to other women, showing them hope and a way forward. I can say to mothers, "I remember that dark place where you are now, and here I am." Let's all ask ourselves, How do we honor these precious angels when their lives, although lost, had purpose? Whether it was one day, three weeks, six months, a year, or sixteen years … Thanks to my son, I understand the value of life. Leveraging the loss clarifies its purpose.

And so, this was the lived-in experience I put behind my doctoral degree. Howard and Mom were still guiding me.

After conquering the skeleton in the closet, I assumed I'd continue as a Michigan State nursing administrator and faculty member. I was serving as the Director of Student Affairs and was responsible for the admissions of nursing students. A colleague asked me to write a National Institutes of Health supplement on her existing grant to investigate more closely the pregnancy outcomes of Black and Latinx women. We were funded, and that outcome shifted my trajectory. The dean advised that I transition out of my administrative role. "You're an NIH-funded researcher now." She asked if I wanted a tenure-track position. I said sure, figuring I'd live out my career on a research faculty at a Big Ten university!

Yet again, the journey took me elsewhere. Trust the process and enjoy the journey, especially the unexpected turns.

> *In their hearts humans plan their course, but*
> *the Lord establishes their steps*
>
> **—PROVERBS 16:9 NIV**

Public health came calling again, disrupting my academic appointment, which offered summers off, in the form of a deputy health officer position at the Ingham County Health Department. I was recruited back because they wanted to steep *health equity and social justice action* into all they did as a department and build a groundbreaking model for how public health should operate.

My second act in public health practice opened several doors, including national recognition and partnerships due to our accomplishments in applying facilitated dialogue as a strategy to achieve health equity and social justice. Others flocked to our work because of its authenticity and transparency—backed by conviction and a desire to create change. From this chapter of my life, the equity leadership principles that I share in *Room at the Table* were born.

Today, I serve as the CEO of the Michigan Public Health Institute (MPHI), a nationally engaged institute headquartered in Okemos, Michigan. I also serve on the faculty of the Charles Stewart Mott Department of Public Health in the College of Medicine at Michigan State University. My commitment to justice and health equity stems from my progressively building experiences along with subsequent and continuous introspections. Soon, I'll invite you to begin a parallel process yourself.

Introspections … My life's work has been aligned in so many ways. I can't help but see the signs! The "Tuskegee Study of Untreated Syphilis in the Negro Male" was relatively overlooked until more recent attention in the field. The ordeal occurred between 1932 and 1972, condoned by the United States Public Health Service and the Centers for Disease Control and Prevention (CDC). In this study, the effects of untreated syphilis were observed in four hundred Black men. These men were unaware of the nature of the experiment and left ignorant when penicillin was developed as an effective treatment. Many died, and legacies were lost.

I thought I was thoroughly familiar with this study until one of my colleagues shared an original publication. I had read other publications from the 1930s. Still, this shared PDF struck me at a new level when I read the title: "Control of Syphilis in a Southern Rural Area: A Preliminary Report" by L. E. Burney, MD, past assistant surgeon of the US Public Health Service, in Brunswick, Georgia.

What hit me in the gut was that this atrocity took place not only in Tuskegee, Alabama, but also at another large site in Brunswick, Georgia, where my family lived. My mother, father, grandmothers, and extended family … *Brunswick*. My family vacations, beach trips, crab fests—Brunswick. This racist public health disaster began the same year my father was born. They were knocking on people's doors and trying to get teachers, ministers, and preachers to push people to participate in the forty-year study. The test subjects were likely associates, and friends, relatives of my father, uncles, and grandfather—probably other relatives, their friends, their church leaders, alas, their community.

Brunswick is a fairly small, predominantly African American community. Looking at the PDF, I saw that everything about it hit too close to home, figuratively and actually, including the reprehensible things said about Brunswick and its residents as seen through the white researcher's lens! How I wish I had learned this truth sooner so I could ask my grandmother, with all her wit and popularity, about what went on. But as I write from my eighty-eight-year-old father's room in a rehab center in North Carolina, I managed to catch him in between doses of medication and told him this story. He cleared his throat and said, "Well, I'm not surprised a bit," and turned to continue his nap. Suddenly, Dr. King's words that "we are caught in an inescapable network of mutuality" resonated for me without question. How could I possibly have a direct or even a close indirect relationship to this historic study? The continuing need for action seems clear across time and generations.

But if racism could have been easily fixed by Black people, we would've checked that box a long time ago. The same is likely true for all marginalized communities. It takes partnership and collaboration among us all to reverse these historic wrongs. We were *created* to be in relationships with one another. I take on racism because I am relationship driven, and racism damages relationships. The solution is not simple. Indeed it is greater and deeper than the flawed mantra to treat everyone the same.

> **equality:**
> *the state of being equal, especially in status, rights, and opportunities.*
>
> **equity:**
> *the policy or practice of accounting for the differences in each individual's starting point when pursuing a goal or achievement, and working to remove barriers to equal opportunity, as by providing support based upon the unique needs of individuals.*

This book is not about equality. We are not equal. *Room at the Table* presents the principles of *equity* so that you can better understand yourself, and understand others, as we strive to make a lasting difference in this world. None of us has come from the same place. We must learn to *acknowledge* difference and not dismiss it. You'll be encouraged to tap into your personal stories and lived experiences to better see opportunities and spaces where privilege, or the lack thereof, has shaped your *thinking, seeing, and doing*. You'll explore health disparities and inequities. No, it's not an easy journey. *Ultimately, our tests become testimonies, and our trials can set the trail for our triumph and journey to victory.*

At the end of each chapter, I'll ask you to reflect. I was once asked as a panel participant, "Can you give us *lessons learned*?" As you'll come to understand after chapter 1, I offer that these are less past-tense events and more actively *learning lessons* because the action is ongoing—we're continuing to grow, deepen, understand, and push forward. As equity leaders, lessons continuously teach us. They remain active. The "Learning Lessons" in this book are the manageable nuggets/chunks/tidbits of content that provoke our thinking. They are the aha moments that reoccur at the most opportune time, advancing our ideas and actions.

I'll also invite you to engage in introspection through our "Mirror Moments," questions that challenge you to pull out that mirror, look yourself in the eye, and forge a deeper understanding of equity and yourself. Though I'm coming from academia (and still in it!), I don't want you to memorize this work. I want you to *internalize* it. I'm speaking to your head, but more importantly, I'm speaking to your heart. Remember—who you are is as important as what you do, if not more so! What stories are you bringing to the table?

> ULTIMATELY, OUR TESTS BECOME TESTIMONIES, AND OUR TRIALS CAN SET THE TRAIL FOR OUR TRIUMPH AND JOURNEY TO VICTORY.

On your mark, get set, reflect!

LEARNING LESSONS: INTRODUCTION

- We all have reflective realizations.
- Equity is not equality.
- Wherever you go, there you are; your lived experiences guide your journey.

MIRROR MOMENTS: INTRODUCTION

1. What is your earliest memory of race?
2. Think about your social identities—your race, ethnicity, class, gender, and others. Which of these shape your day-to-day actions most predominately?
3. Was the race memory question easy to respond to? Was the identity question easy to respond to? Why or why not?

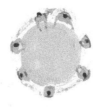

CHAPTER ONE

LEADERING—EQUITY IN MOTION

> **leader:**
>
> *noun: the person who leads or commands a group, organization, or country. verb: ???*

I'm a lover of words, and the term *leadering* popped into my mind one day. I was reflecting on the words *lead*, *leader*, and *leading*. I thought to myself, *Wait!* Most words that end in *–er* suggest action. A helper is someone who is helping, a teacher is someone who is teaching, and a preacher is someone who is preaching. But something distinct happens with the word *leader*. We don't often say that a leader is someone who is leading; rather, "leader" is a label. A professional gets dubbed a leader, and it's a noun for who they *are*, not what they're *doing*. Being a leader is a fixed term—not in motion—and then it occurred to me that the term *leadering* is perhaps the action. It's continuous. Leadering isn't stagnant. *I'm teaching, I'm helping, I'm* *preaching*, or *I'm leadering*. The equity leader that I am is continuous, and it must hold the same for you.

There's much to learn about being an effective leader and plenty of books on the subject. How do you hold space in a room? How do you set a culture, climate, and context in which people can be their best selves? My approach to equity leadership suggests, *I'm going to hold space with you, I'll make room at the table, and I will do this continuously*. Not because I have a title. Rather, I have a commitment to advancing change and seeing that *together* we accomplish something. I never get to check the box: "I'm a leader." When I'm no longer leadering, I'm no longer fulfilling my position for equity change.

I'm a singer. Whether I'm singing or not at this moment, I'm still a singer. I'm a follower of Christ; no matter where I am, I'm still a follower. I'm a leader; whether I'm leadering or not at this moment, I'm a leader. It is a presence. A leader's soul has a lens that captures what's happening all around them. I always peer through an equity lens because what I've seen in this life can't be unseen. My equity lens comprises the conceptual models and practices that shape my worldview and priorities in centering equity to advance change. No one chooses their talent or calling; it often chooses them. My experience and studies, my understanding of history, my view of this world as a Black woman, and my calling and purpose allow me to bring my full self to equity leadership.

THE PATRIOT—THE SERVANT—THE EQUITY LEADER

*The servant-leader is servant first. It begins with the
natural feeling that one wants to serve, to serve first.
Then conscious choice brings one to aspire to lead.*

—ROBERT K. GREENLEAF

My job isn't possible without recognizing the impact of power. How do I leverage and apply more effectively the impact of power in alignment with equity principles? This is very different from "I'm the boss. My way or the highway." No, how do I *use* power in respect to others? I'm inspired by the servant-leadership model. Greenleaf's work is groundbreaking, but it's just the beginning. You *can* be a servant leader without attending to the issues of race and oppression. We are focusing on a different model of leadership—the *future* model.

Yes, I'm a servant leader, but I am bound to go beyond that. I'm an *equity* leader. Today's leaders need to talk about what it means to equitably cocreate—to unlearn so many traditions. Think of the clichés: "It's lonely at the top" and "That's why you get paid the big bucks." These sorts of statements and paradigms are what make leaders think they are singularly the expositors of what will drive the best interests of those in the workforce or organization.

I intentionally rid myself of old paradigms and step into new territory. Equity leadership requires innovation. I must admit when *I don't know what I don't know*. Perhaps the one who knows what I don't know is *you*. I oversee a workforce that I'm privileged to lead. I'm honored to guide them, just as I trust they'll guide me in return. I've had to unprogram many leadership stereotypes, and so have my colleagues. We're in this together.

There has been quite a bit of pushback, if not backlash, against leading through an equity lens. Of all the assumptions out there, I'm struck by a tendency to correlate equity leadership with a lack of patriotism, as the title of this section suggests. Certainly not everything in these United States in which I've lived, loved, and learned is wrong. I believe in the promise of this country. My father and brother are veterans who served our nation. Having been raised in a culture of patriotism, I know that equity leadership is not *un*patriotic; rather, it is asking ourselves, "Are we the best we can be right now?" I don't think anyone can say, "Yes, we're the best we can be right now."

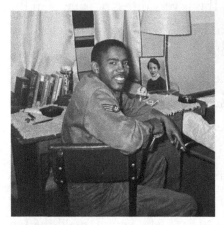 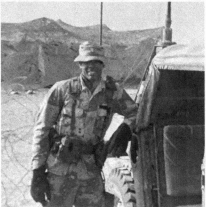

Left: My father, twenty-three-year veteran, then Airman 1st Class, John W. Branch II
Right: My brother, then 1st Lt. Gary Branch, USMA Class of 1988

We get comfortable in the space of *good enough*. Well, good enough isn't good enough! I'll keep reminding you of this … It's not good enough because we can do better as a community—better as a nation. We can hold up the principles that our men and women in uniform fight for.

As a sociologist, I often refer to the work of Gunnar Myrdal. In 1944, he wrote *An American Dilemma: The Negro Problem and Modern Democracy*. He noted that we as Americans say the right things—we recite the Pledge of Allegiance and have a sound constitution. "We hold these truths to be self-evident, that all men are created equal …" But *An American Dilemma* noted the contradiction that most of this isn't true in the lived experiences of so many Americans. What does it truly mean to say, "With liberty and justice for all?" *What does that mean?* As an equity leader, I don't see it taking place.

How can we reconcile that there are inconsistencies there? Because there *are* inconsistencies and contradictions. Equity leadership actively seeks out what's unfair. It's not just about going to your job and getting the work done. If something occurs that is unfair, then your job is to do something about it. Seek it out, not for the sake of observation but for the sake of reversing, amending, changing, challenging, revising, and *healing* it. Unfairness isn't about inequality; it's about inequity.

There are some things that you just don't see—until you do. We'll discuss this occurrence in chapter 4, but for now, allow me to share what I call my Chevy Cavalier phenomenon. When my oldest son was in high school, I knew I needed to find a little knockabout car for him. One of my friends suggested, "Oh, the Detroit city government is auctioning their fleet. They have a bunch of Chevy Cavaliers. We could get you a ticket to the auction." I had to ask, "What's a Chevy Cavalier?" So I went online and looked it up. Sure enough, it was a great little knockabout car. We go to the auction, get the car, and I'm driving the Cavalier home. I'm telling you, on that day, everybody must have realized that Cavaliers were on sale because I saw them all over the place! In truth, there were just a ton of these cars out there on the streets already, but I didn't see it until I saw it.

No one owns Black people as property today; we all eat in the same restaurants and go to the same schools (for the most part). We've come far and can be tempted now to leave good enough alone. *No, we can't!* Because our grandchildren should inherit a country that stands truer to what the founders of this nation suggested. Let's actively engage to claim the original spirit and intent of our country—the bedrock of its soul. And let's be honest, in my field, it is about saving lives. For this to happen, we need equity leaders like you.

Grassroots versus grass-tops advocacy is a classic paradigm that I'd like to agitate.[1] It always struck me that we don't say *grassroots versus grass shoots*. Grassroots and grass tops seems odd—mostly because it doesn't rhyme like grassroots and grass shoots—and also because we fail to see the connectedness of the root to the shoot. You can't have grass shooting out of the ground without it being connected to the root. The grass top does not exist without the root and the shoot that connects them. This point reiterates the fact that, as an equity leader, you're not a grass top! *Look at me, I get all the attention up here*. No. Don't forget why you get to be up there. You are positioned to do the work in connection with the roots. Your strength comes from the root to the shoot. Never forget that.

GRAPPLING: A NECESSARY INGREDIENT

grapple:

to engage in a close fight or struggle without weapons; wrestle.

I discovered early on as a new CEO at MPHI that I was the culture broker and vision caster for the organization. Working toward health equity, social justice, antiracism, and antioppression is hard, but it taught me that *where we grapple is where we grow*. To grapple is to struggle, and this is where the greatest rewards await us. The idiom "the struggle is real" invites levity to the weightiness of this truth. Grappling is necessary to unearth the inequities that

FAITH TO CHANGE, FAITH TO GRAPPLE, FAITH TO HEAL—ALL OF THESE ARE PROFOUND REWARDS FOR HARD WORK.

---

1   Mukundan Sivaraj, "Grasstops vs. Grassroots and Why You Should Combine Both," CallHub, June 26, 2020, https://callhub.io/grasstops-vs-grassroots/.

challenge the well-being of so many. These inequities often seem impossible to overcome, but I am fully persuaded that it is worth the grappling. *Faith to change, faith to grapple, faith to heal—all of these are profound rewards for hard work.*

In launching our health equity workshop in Ingham County, it was interesting to observe that the people who were most resistant or hesitant (i.e., they were grappling) were those who emailed me months later to say, "I'm so glad you required us to do this workshop." They didn't know what they didn't know—didn't see it till they saw it—and grappling revealed this to them.

At these workshops, there was *much* grappling to face. The counternarrative sounded like this: "She's making us do this class, and it's terrible"—most commonly from white colleagues fearing they would be attacked. They found the idea to be almost terrifying at first. But then they'd reach out after day two, asking, "Has the workshop changed?" No, it was the same. To their surprise, after day two, they didn't feel attacked at all. Our intent was never to attack. That isn't how we do our work. Our intent is to *keep people whole and keep people at the table.* That became our ongoing mantra and my continuing philosophy for how to advance this work.

I'm not trying to convince or persuade anyone that I'm right and they're wrong about inequity. Leadering—that continuous process—incites dialogue as often as possible. Grappling together, we initiate a shared experience that we all have together—that we all crave. Through this process, we transform lives and futures. To do this, to initiate grappling as an equity leader, you can't be a stagnant leader content with your big office. You need action. I define leadering as the *praxis* of leadership. Praxis is the integration of theory and practice—it requires reflection and a com-

KEEP PEOPLE WHOLE AND KEEP PEOPLE AT THE TABLE.

mitment to the *practical*. While servant leadership has an unspoken focus on those being led, *leadering* requires self-reflection and a commitment to *doing*. That's a praxis!

> **praxis:**
> *practice, as distinguished from theory.*
> *praxis = (reflection + action) + change.*

Nobody wants to grapple. As we'll discuss in chapter 2, no one wants to wake up in the morning feeling outraged by what they see in the world. But we must grapple to disrupt the status quo. Within equity dialogues, you begin to recognize when something is completely off track. You get comfortable in your gut, in your heart, in your head, and in your ability to call out—in a way that deconstructs old habits—inequitable systems built into our society.

I read once that FBI agents who do counterfeit work don't study the counterfeit dollars; they study the *real* dollar bills. It's the same principle in equity leadership. Have a keen vision and a laser-focused mind on what *should be* instead of what shouldn't. You can't just say, "That was racist," "That was homophobic," or "That was ageist or ableist." No … What is the thing that *should* be? When you get in sync with that, anything that contradicts it raises a flag. This process is not about blame, shame, or attack. We all want to be led toward a different space. Not the counterfeit, but the real.

Sure, the world has changed … a little bit. We are still living with the residual consequences of deeply planned and strategized actions: gender oppression, class discrimination, and racism. They remain steeped in our society. *Just ignore it. It'll go away.* I think not! Ignore it and it will continue to have the negative consequences that it was designed to have. Equity leadership sets a vision for that affirming, seeing-oriented, hearing-oriented, active healing space that cultivates our best and healthiest selves, and anything that contradicts this gives us permission to deconstruct, unpack, and reframe. Because we're in a place where we just want to pretend as though we've arrived when we have not. We're not our best selves yet!

Do we want ourselves to be at our best? Note the collective pronoun *ourselves*. It's about doing this together. Charles-Edward Amory Winslow, an early twentieth-century American bacteriologist and public health expert, talks about the mission of public health to be what we as a society do *together* to assure the conditions needed for good health. I would submit that anything we do together requires *equity*. We can't do it together if there's not enough room at the table.

In my equity teaching, people want to argue that the issues I present aren't about race; they're about economics—*people are poor, so it's not about them being Black, Brown, or Latinx, etc.* But we also know from research methodology and analysis in sociology that even when we can control for race in our studies, there is still what we call an *unexplained variance*. I love this phrase.

variance:
the fact or quality of being different, divergent, or inconsistent.

There is something we still can't explain that differentiates the experiences of white people from those of Black and Brown people (BIPOC). We believe that this unexplained variance is measuring *racism* and how the color of our skin manifests and guides the lives that we live. It is comfortable to argue that this variance pertains to economics because talking about racism, let alone *deconstructing* racism, is hard. And yet, as my students have witnessed, that facilitated dialogue frees people and creates interpersonal connections. We begin to see one another …

I'm not an archaeologist, but I love to watch the History Channel programs about digs where ancient societies are unearthed and discovered. I'm in awe when the History Channel archaeologist comes in, starts digging, and realizes, "Wow, there's this whole city under there!" Further still, the fact that old societies even exist under new societies has the potential for contemporary negative consequences. Maybe it's a sinkhole, a structural problem for new buildings, the construction is shifting and off kilter, or perhaps there's an unusual element tainting the soil. The unseen, *unexplained variance*. There are still *consequences* from the past.

That's exactly where I believe we are as a society. Equity leaders are cultural archeologists. We're starting to unmask some things that are uncomfortable. We're grappling, and that's okay. When we unearth traumatizing systems, we *act*—we study their existence and recognize what contributes to the negative impact. Because of this, our positioning as equity leaders has the potential to change many lives.

> **EQUITY LEADERSHIP— AND I TELL THIS TO MY MENTEES—IS NOT ABOUT THE POSITION; IT IS ABOUT THE POSITIONING.**

POSITIONING TO LEAD—LEADING TO POSITION

> *As some wise person said, It's not that you need to think less of yourself, it's that you need to think of yourself less.*
>
> —CELESTE GIORDANO

As my career advanced, and I'll say, in my time of quiet, meditative prayer, I had an epiphany. *Equity leadership—and I tell this to my mentees—is not about the position; it is about the positioning.* Dare I say, equity leadership has an awareness of *positionality* and the questionable positions life has put us in. We are invited into rooms that we might not otherwise have been invited into before. We have vantage points that we previously did not have. We have an advantage or privilege to now *act* in a way that blesses, helps, and redirects others. It's not about the position or the title; it's about our own *positioning* and how we utilize that positioning to become a force for change.

EQUITY LEADERSHIP TYPOLOGY

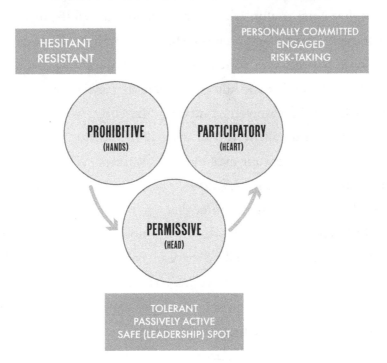

I have observed the manifestation of *positionality* in three typologies of leadership: prohibitive, permissive, or participatory. These typologies are shaped by the leaders' engagement with their staff. The prohibitive leader is just that—*No, we can't do **that*** (i.e., say "racism," talk about diversity … choose your definition for "that"). The permissive leader initially gives a favorable response—*Go ahead, yes. Go for it.* And then the catch follows—*But don't call on me; you've got it, go ahead.* Last, there is the participatory leader—fully engaged, supportive, and advocating. *Let's do this together; what do you need from me?* These typologies either disable, enable, or equip. I've observed the pattern over and over in diverse organizations and agencies.

I am advocating for equity-focused participatory leadership, but I would also submit (on top of that) that in our society, leadership must be adaptive and intuitive. It must actually transcend helpful typologies. I can't speak to everyone in the room like they're the same person. It is naive to think that we can deconstruct all the hierarchies and become a matrix organization where each individual is the same, allowing us to proclaim, "Here's how it goes!" It doesn't work that way.

None of this is easy, but even when we can't fully *deconstruct* a hierarchy, we can evolve to function differently. As we are transitioning, we can do all we can to work better within the hierarchy. That means keeping your eyes open at all times. Whenever there's something that suggests, *This is the way it's been done for years*, then X marks the spot. You can guarantee that a protocol in place for twenty years highlights inequity at work. I love Simon Sinek's admonition on finding your *why*: "Let us all be the leaders we wish we had." That's a *why* for me. It gives me the courage to fully engage and do hard things—fully see within and across the hierarchical systems in place.

I remember a particularly tough day on the job when there was tension and interpersonal clashing. Someone asked aloud, "Why bother? This is so hard. Let's just get as much done as we can and stop trying to do this deeper 'equity work'!" *Why bother* ... I couldn't help but extend Sinek's words about the power of *why*. Indeed, "Find your *why* and lose your *why bother*." *Why bother* is self-talk combined with external chatter that will convince you to not do the hard equity-centered work or drop the heavy lift for change. *Why bother* is the phrase of exasperation muttered as you throw in the towel or give up. There can't be a *why bother* in public health. Lives depend upon us holding firm. Embrace your *why* and resist the temptation to give up. You've been positioned to help, to bless, to change, and to lead.

Because this work is hard, you as the leader must make room at the table, invite and welcome others—keeping them at the table. I'm also a fan of *The Five Love Languages*, by Gary Chapman. As a leader, I am *other* focused, striving to figure out the love languages or needs of others with whom I work or partner ... Maybe it's just the recognition and celebration of what someone did. Maybe it's quality time, like grabbing lunch together. Perhaps it's a day off. Our team has been discussing the work-life balance a lot lately. Many are working from home. But what does *work-life balance* even mean?

The myth of the professional self versus the personal self is an antagonist of equity leadership. I share my journey and stories in this book to invite you to be similarly vulnerable and transparent as leaders. Perhaps some of these stories make you say to yourself, *I remember when something like that happened to me!* There will be moments of grappling as you peer through the equity lens. We see things not as *they* are but as *we* are (a statement I make often that is also a quote attributed to Anaïs Nin). So when we expand our view of humanity by sharing and hearing what others have gone through, we begin to *see, say, and do differently*. That's how we move humanity forward.

PRO:

Latin: In front of, before.

PER:

Latin: Through, during.

The truth is that you can't separate your work life from your personal life—not as an equity leader. My home life influences my thoughts at work, and my work life influences my attitudes when home. Why do we try to disconnect these? And how do we permit ourselves to be authentic in what we do? You can't tell me, "This isn't personal; it's professional." This *is* personal. It *all* is. In my role, people trust me to carry out my work in a way that will be healing—keeping people's wholeness intact while also *increasing* their wholeness.

As a senior equity leader, if you're not focused on making people whole, your team won't do as well, and the outcomes, products, services, or *change* that you provide to the community will never reach their potential. There **must** be willingness and full investment for the long haul. *Leadering*—equity leadership in motion … There's no conclusion to what we do.

LEARNING LESSONS: LEADERING

- Leadering is an action—an ever-flowing, ever-going drive for change.
- We grow where we grapple.
- Servant leadership is the building block for equity leadership.
- It's not about the position; it's about the positioning.

MIRROR MOMENTS: LEADERING

1. What are three adjectives that come to mind when you think of an equity leader?
2. What is the overlap between who you are as a leader and how you perceive equity leaders?
3. Have you observed a leader who rested on their laurels? Was it justified or problematic? Why or why not?

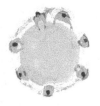

CHAPTER TWO

PRODUCTIVE OUTRAGE

It is necessary that the weakness of the powerless is transformed into a force capable of announcing justice. For this to happen, a total denouncement of fatalism is necessary. We are transformative beings and not beings for accommodation.

—PAULO FREIRE

I n 2018, I was working on a concept for a grant focusing on maternal health—and particularly maternal death—that would center the role of leaders in the field. My three colleagues in the room shared a lot of angst. *Why aren't maternal-health leaders doing more? Why aren't they leveraging their power and influence as directors, presidents, vice presidents, and CEOs to make meaningful change? Why are so many okay with the status quo?* Out of our discussions came the phrase *productive outrage*. That's it—we need more *productive outrage*!

Righteous indignation is a term that many have heard … It's the cousin of productive outrage. Let's focus on the *productive* part of the phrase. Righteous indignation and productive outrage are two phrases that represent different schools of thought, or mental models, expressing a response to something frustrating and maddening, albeit using different semantics. What do we do with the anger that ensues? Anger is a great fuel for action, but we must choose to have it fuel the *right* action. There is no use in challenging inequity if our actions are destructive. Anger can fuel terrible, wrong, or harmful outcomes. Instead, let it fuel *productive* outrage. Don't tell yourself how terrible something is without committing to act constructively in response.

> HOW WILL YOUR OUTRAGE—THAT HIGHER INDIGNATION—CAUSE YOU TO SAY, "NOPE, I CAN'T TAKE IT ANYMORE. I HAVE TO STAND UP AND ACT. I HAVE TO DO SOMETHING!"

The Black community feels outraged when they see yet another Black man or woman killed in a police-involved shooting. Other communities—Asian, Latinx, and LGBTQ+—feel rage when their communities are harmed at the hand of injustice. There's *outrage* when we see one more mass shooting in a school or church. You hear it everywhere: "This is so terrible." "This is so upsetting and distressing." Yes, you're expressing your hurt and outrage, but not *productively*. What are you going to *do*? *How will your outrage—that higher indignation—cause you to say, "Nope, I can't take it anymore. I have to stand up and act. I have to do something!"*

Outrage can lead to backlash. Productive outrage is indignation that drives sustained change. Productive outrage leads to action, and vigilance through discourse. So, let's have a dialogue.

DIALOGUE AS ACTION

> *Change happens by listening and then starting a dialogue with the people who are doing something you don't believe is right.*
>
> —JANE GOODALL

After the mass shooting in Buffalo, New York, where ten Black men were killed and two injured, my staff asked me to write a statement of sympathy to be posted on our website. I told them flat out, "I'm sick and tired of writing statements." I refused to be a part of another written declaration because all I could think of were the numerous statements published and disseminated after the summer of social unrest after the murder of George Floyd in 2020. What *action* came from those statements? Not much … In many ways, it seemed that organizations just wanted an announcement on their websites to say, "Look, we're a part of the *good* people—we did a statement. That's good, isn't it?"

I'm sorry. No statements. No idle words. Instead, let's think about a tangible action, and if you don't know what to do, the first step is *to have a dialogue.* Initiate three meaningful, action-oriented dialogues with different colleagues or loved ones. (Why three dialogues? It gives you a goal of continuous forward movement. If the first one is awkward, you can't quit—you committed to at least a couple more.) Ask yourself, *What would it look like for us to respond in a way that honors the humanity of ourselves and others?* My words persuaded my staff. I advised that we should all keep thinking—keep the intentional dialogue going—and ditch the statements. It was a first move …

At a recent medical conference, I began my opening remarks by discussing the SCOTUS and the *Roe v. Wade* leak (as it was at the time). My mind drifted to the Buffalo supermarket shooting. *Then* the shooting at the Taiwanese church in California, and also another police-involved shooting of a Black man in Akron, Ohio. You wake up and there's continually something to respond to, and I would submit it is because not much has changed since George Floyd's death. Inaction comes from focusing only on words—*statements.* We've made statements but done nothing more. It's not good enough to "talk the talk," and our experience with the impact of statements shows us it's also not good enough to "chalk the talk." Rather we must "walk the talk"—action rules the day.

Equity leaders are called on like never before to harness their *productive* outrage, a response that is fueled by feeling. However, we are not taught to embrace our feelings and emotions—certainly not in the leadership space and not in the professional space. Rather, the self-talk comes as *No, keep it together. Be calm, cool, and collected.* But that is not the authentic reaction of our whole selves, is it? We are human beings naturally designed to live our lives with emotions. So why should we pretend that we do not have certain emotions in certain spaces? Why should we take on the pressure of that artificial stance? Instead, we must leverage those feelings to fuel a conviction for change.

Emotions interact. Perhaps you are mad, then you're angry, and ultimately, you're frustrated. When you have joy, you are also more likely to feel hopeful, excited, or energized. How do we get in touch with emotions in a meaningful and constructive way to productively fuel or shape our actions and reflections? A good first step is to sit back, reflect, and resist the urge to ignore your feelings. Know what's going on inside you.

In the face of outrageous instances and the absence of meaningful dialogue, that little knot in the pit of your stomach forms, and you push it down. You say to yourself, *Nope, I'm not supposed to be angry. I'm not supposed to be upset. I'm just going to pretend.* I'm always curious about that sensation when you want to cry and you try not to—how physically painful that can be, that horrible tightness in the throat! Is it telling you that the body feels physical pain when simply not expressing emotions?

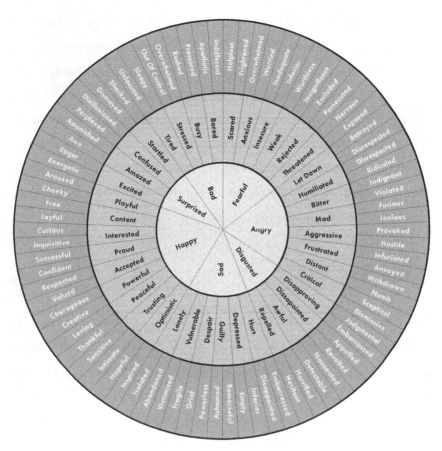

Original source: Dr. Gloria Willcox, "The Feeling Wheel"

Anger might be described as one of the most difficult sensations that we, as humans, can feel. It's considered a "bad" emotion, but in and of itself, it is not. It becomes bad when we allow the feeling to prompt negative or destructive action. Instead, how can we use that energy to *do* something constructive or positive? The Apostle Paul said in Ephesians 4:26, "Be angry but sin not." Once you understand the source of your emotions—often through dialogue with those you trust—you position yourself to find constructive and effective solutions.

I get frustrated (a manifestation of anger) when I see people who are marginalized or treated as *less than*. I get upset when I feel like my voice is excluded. Ahh … the feelings wheel. It has helped me home in on my emotions. Through dialogue—and introspection—we can unpack emotional moments and come up with actionable steps. Productive outrage, righteous indignation, and *just ire* (not used as often)—are all honorable sensations and noble frames for action in very difficult discussions. *Outrage*, *indignation*, and *ire*. Without an adjoining adjective, these reactions can be so destructive, but they can also be profoundly productive as an equity leader when we practice funneling these emotions into change.

PRODUCTIVE CONFLICT

This is what I call sublime (defined as "elevated" and "exalted") ignorance. When many Black people hear stories like this, we do not know whether to scream, cry, or laugh. How could you not know that racism is alive and well in America and throughout the world? The truth is that white people are not required to know. As the dominant group, they can go through life with the privilege of never thinking about their race. Many white people still claim not to "see" race. If you do not see it, there is no reason to address it. You can be sublimely ignorant.

—MARY-FRANCES WINTERS

As the AIDS educator for a joint initiative between the Department of Corrections and the Department of Community Health, I had a rare interaction. I was an employee of the Department of Corrections, and a nurse colleague from the Department of Community Health and I continually butted heads. I consider myself an agreeable and amiable person—easy to get along with—but no matter how I tried, I just did not get along with this guy. No matter what I said, he had a negative and bombastic retort. No matter what I suggested, he would resist and trash the idea. Mind you, he wasn't coming up with anything constructive as an alternative. He also happened to be a yeller! I'd often have to say, "Let's lower our voices ..."

During one of the tense exchanges, I couldn't help but wonder how race and gender might be influencing his continuous negativity, and my outrage was fueled (perhaps not productively). I asked him, "Who do you think you're yelling at?" And before we knew it, we were in the workplace having an all-out yelling match. All I could think was, *Why does this man think he can come at me like this? What is wrong with this guy?* An experience of *destructive* outrage—destructive in that it didn't help the relationship or the work we were responsible for carrying out. The behavior didn't seek to solve the problem. It made me think of Michelle Obama's famous quote, "When they go low, we go high." Well ... he went low, and I followed him right into the pit.

Going high requires a deeper motivation—there needs to be fuel to get us there. This is where productive outrage comes into play and practice. By all means, don't kowtow and submit to the foolishness of others. Address the foolishness constructively. When fueled by rage, you can still make positive change. When something is infuriating—and as an equity leader, you'll experience many such moments—people often don't want to talk about it. If a situation is running hot, there's no need to have *the talk* today, but *not* discussing the incident bypasses an opportunity for growth. Dialogue is action, and people need to constructively express themselves through words in interpersonal relationships.

I serve in a professional group committed to starting a racial-equity journey, and as a gesture in that regard, I took a group on a tour of a historical and well-known plantation. As part of this group excursion, the tour guides were asked to share the history from the perspective of the enslaved people who'd once worked there. Unfortunately, I was unable to participate in the tour but listened as my colleagues processed their experience and reactions after the fact. Many expressed extreme incredulity and disbelief that they weren't taught the behind-the-scenes truths in school!

Yes, I shared my productive outrage in response to their shock. This bit of history seemed obvious … Plantations typically include a beautiful, well-cared-for mansion, but who took care of it? And what must it have been like for the people taking care of it? I found myself feeling the same productive outrage when listening to white Americans on popular genealogy shows expressing distress when they learn that their southern ancestors owned slaves. How could we live our lives as if those things never occurred? We'll be discussing making the invisible visible in chapter 5, but, back to my outrage …

My colleagues were taken aback by my strong and somewhat corrective response, or shall I say, my *retort*. But that is the courageous risk that must be taken to catapult outrage into action. I couldn't sit there and not take advantage of the teachable moment within the discourse. I thanked everyone for sharing their feelings and gave breath to my own feelings, as direct and difficult as those emotions were. It is counterintuitive to say that you want to start an antiracist journey yet be shocked at the evidence of racism. It would seem that it is the evidence of racism that drives us to start an antiracist or antioppression journey.

Productive outrage evolves from a personal reaction to either interpersonal, social, or systemic factors. In this case, my own *Black fatigue* collided with well-meaning yet disingenuous efforts. People of color tire of educating white people about the obvious things happening in our lives. By *our* lives, I don't just mean BIPOC lives but also our collective lives, as events occur in and around white lives as well. My productive outrage pushed me to be disruptive in that situation so that people couldn't go back to their former polite ways of thinking and doing. As equity leaders, we must be open to the candor and risk of allowing strong emotions to shape powerful, effective, authentic, and *active* responses.

Equity leadership is a transformative pursuit—it creates space for otherwise unheard voices to be heard—even outraged voices. There may likely be backlash. No one wants to be labeled, and remaining quiet is often a type of protective strategy. When you express yourself and get discounted with words like "There they go again …" then leaning into productive outrage becomes *even more* essential. When we find ourselves as equity leaders in marginalized positions, it's crucial to own our emotions and use them in a way that advances change and shores up relationships. It's safer and easier to *not bother*, but this tendency blocks collective and mutual growth. As a side note: yes, choose your battles; be strategic. *Your productive outrage has value and sometimes that outrage manifests in strategic silence.* Believe me, the opportunity to engage will always present itself again.

The fear of being stigmatized often stifles. Thus I often ask myself, *How do we push and prod people in these equity-driven spaces? How do we push them to see and speak? And once we get people to speak their truths, how do we deal with the natural reactions?* Outrage *is* a natural reaction to racialized and gender-driven occurrences. First of all, this outrage must be heard and acknowledged, and second of all, *how do we make it productive for change?*

I consider myself a happy and content person, and I'd love to be that way all the time! I can only imagine how, in the civil rights era, activists were thinking they'd

> **YOUR PRODUCTIVE OUTRAGE HAS VALUE AND SOMETIMES THAT OUTRAGE MANIFESTS IN STRATEGIC SILENCE.**

rather not risk the attacks of dogs and fire hoses but instead remain content and at peace. The weight that we carry seems far less than the weight placed on those who went before us. When we disrupt a moment, we put a dent in a legacy of pain, silence, and swallowed outrage. Today, we are in a space to use our outrage for change. Equity leaders continuously hold space for these moments. So whether you are happy and content, or serious and impatient, take a deep breath. Don't hold it in, but exhale and use it for what must be done.

PRODUCTIVE VIGILANCE

Eternal vigilance is the price of liberty, and it does seem to me that notwithstanding all these social agencies and activities there is not that vigilance which should be exercised in the preservation of our rights.

—IDA B. WELLS-BARNETT

One of the biggest enemies of equity is the loss of vigilance. During the AIDS epidemic, we had such huge advances, and so we hit a point in the trajectory of the epidemic where things were improving. For *young* gay men, although in proximity to HIV and AIDS, the epidemic was considered "old-school stuff." The younger community worried less about the virus. It seemed there was an attitude of *That was y'all, and this is us* … During this era of complacency,[2] we began to see the numbers go up in the wrong direction.

The same lack of vigilance was seen in syphilis. As the local health officer, I recall the unexpected appearance at my office door of the communicable disease nurse late on a Friday afternoon. I always joked, "Public health crises only start on Fridays." In this exchange, I was handed a fax that had just come in (yes, important public health information came through a fax machine then). It was a communicable disease report stating that there was a new case of syphilis. I had

---

2   Centers for Disease Control and Prevention, "Diagnoses of HIV Infection in the United States and Dependent Areas, 2019," *HIV Surveillance Report 2021*, 32.

to ask, "Do they mean *syphilis* syphilis? Or do they mean gonorrhea?" No, it was syphilis. The syphilis numbers had dropped significantly for an extended time frame, and so this new case was highly concerning. I've seen the same thing happen with measles after the numbers go down, and with mumps.

As I write this, there was a 2022 case of polio reported in New York. The bugs are doing what the bugs do … Everyone thought polio was "gone," but it wasn't. The science of vaccinations provided a population protection, and in vaccinations' absence, and because of other public health strategies, numbers revert. The things that resulted in decreased numbers must be sustained to keep numbers down. Complacency and loss of vigilance cause us to let our guards down. We arguably must apply similar vigilance as we strive to maintain the decreasing spread of COVID-19.

I use these public health problems as an example, highlighting a larger point. When we lose vigilance as equity leaders, we start to see things returning to what I would describe as chaos. Public health and equity leadership are not check-the-box pursuits. They are continuous actions (leadering) that move toward finding a solution and then maintaining the solution over time.

Productive outrage and vigilance go hand in hand. They drive one another. It's true, outrage is a strong emotion. I don't wake up in the morning asking myself, *When can I experience outrage today?* In all fairness, I'd prefer an outrage-free day … I want the day to be peaceful, calm, and joyful. This is where vigilance comes into play—keeping things going in the right direction so that productive outrage isn't spent in vain. It fuels us forward.

Be angry and do not sin; do not let the sun go down on your anger.

—EPHESIANS 4:26

LEARNING LESSONS: PRODUCTIVE OUTRAGE

- Dialogue is doing.
- Outrage is destructive, but productive outrage is constructive and transformative.
- Equity leadership requires vigilance. We're focused on continuous action for change.
- Reject the "check a box" leadership mentality.

MIRROR MOMENTS: PRODUCTIVE OUTRAGE

1. Reflect on two circumstances: when frustration caused you to shut down and when it inspired you to act. What was the difference in those instances?
2. Can you describe a time when you saw someone treated poorly because of their race, class, gender, or another identity? How did the incident affect you? How did you respond, or how could you have responded?
3. How can you cultivate the courage to respond to outrageous and racialized incidents?

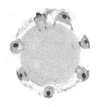

CHAPTER THREE

THINKING DIFFERENTLY

Hear no evil, see no evil, speak no evil.

*An instruction to avoid bad behavior, this expression is now often used
to mean to ignore bad behavior by pretending not to hear or see it.*

—MACMILLAN DICTIONARY

W hen I started my public health career in HIV work in 1987,
there was a young white boy in a rural community who con-
tracted the virus. The health officer called me in and said,
"Hey, we have a situation. The public is panicking. The school is
panicking. Just set up a community meeting for them ..."

I was saying to myself, *Uh, okay?* I had some concerns, but still,
I had a job to do, so I started making calls, trying to figure things
out. I worked out the logistics—whether we should hold this at the
public library or perhaps a local church. I checked our health officer's
calendar. This was my first professional job, and I assumed he would

be there for such high-stakes conversation, so of course I would need his support and attendance …

I arranged everything, scheduled the gathering for the following week, and then reported back to the health officer. "We're all set. I found a location. Your calendar is clear, and we're all good to go." He asked why I checked his calendar. That question rang as oddly as his prior statement for me to *just* set up a community meeting! When I responded that I wanted to make sure he was available, he reminded me that I was the AIDS educator and not him.

Now I was the one panicking. *You cannot possibly be sending me to a hysteria-stricken rural white community!* Here I am, reverting in my mind to the little Black girl who had sandwiches packed during family road trips. Any Black leader, let alone a Black female leader reading this, likely knows what I'm talking about.

I had to ask myself, "How can I increase comfort with discomfort? How do I resist impostor syndrome, especially when complicated through race and difference?" That's the very work of equity leadership—stepping into discomfort to create comfort (you'll hear about my blue jeans analogy soon). Anyhow, I was panicking but determined, and my health officer just kind of smiled and told me that I was excellent at my job. That didn't make the anxiety go away. But—*deep breath*—I knew I had to do it.

On the day of the meeting, I headed to this small rural community. Upon arrival, I introduced myself and gave my AIDS 101 debrief based on the facts as we knew them at that time. I will submit that we didn't know a lot about AIDS at that early stage. Even with my small bank of knowledge, I knew more than they did, and what they wanted was not necessarily a bunch of facts—they needed someone to hear their pain, fears, worries, and concerns. Most of my responses at that community meeting involved listening, thinking, and self-reflection on what was the right thing to say. How could I appropriately use the knowledge that I'd gained—going to conferences, reading articles—so that it would affirm their concerns and help *reframe* their concerns and feelings through the facts?

Lo and behold, my health officer's confidence in me was not misplaced. It was a successful session. Over this hour-and-a-half meeting, and staying after to talk to the people who lingered behind, I found myself moving from "I have to do this" to "I want to do this. I want to help people understand." Driving home, I thought about how I *get* to make a difference in people's lives. It was amazing!

This epiphany came with a lot of emotional and intellectual angst—panic, concern, and self-doubt. Sure, I could have just gone in there with an expert attitude and said, "Okay, everybody sit down. I have information, the facts ... I have some flip charts for you, and here we go. Just listen to what I have to say." I wasn't yet the equity leader that I am today (primarily because we didn't use that term!), but this experience was a great lesson for the leader that I would become ... am *still* becoming.

I began to think differently.

HUMILITY—CHOOSING TO THINK DIFFERENTLY

humility:

a modest or low view of one's own importance; humbleness.

You can't be an equity leader without humility. It is the very nature of the leadership style I am recommending to you. I learned a valuable lesson during that community discussion because I discovered quickly that more than anything, the people in attendance wanted me to hold space with them. I often look back on that incident and have to ask myself, "Would I have trusted a brand new employee to do what I did?" I mean, that was a high-risk, high-stakes event!

My health officer could have legitimately taken the lead in this community meeting, even if he had me attend for subject expertise, but he didn't. Because he didn't, I am challenged over thirty years after the event to demonstrate such leadership courage. The easy path is *discomfort avoidance*. "If it's not comfortable, simply don't let them do it. Handle it yourself." I am more grateful for that experience now as a senior leader than I was as a new line staff. I was scared, but I had the privilege to step into my fear and help others.

"Thinking differently" is about *getting* to do the important things. Leadership can often be about *shoulds* or *wants*, and we can get stuck there. *I guess I want to do this …* etc. Many, many leaders, whether they are willing to admit to it or not, are in the stalled position of "Do we have to? Do we have to enter difficult moments or conversations—even if they are ultimately *transcending* moments—for the sake of equity and humility?"

Equity-driven leadership prompts us to challenge the authenticity of our thoughts. Some may think they have to adhere to a new protocol, or if they say certain words enough, they will appear to do the right thing. And then perhaps the grappling, the problem under the surface, will just go away. Not likely. Going from *I have to* to *I want to* to *I get to* is an intentional choice. Each transition and movement is intentional and reinforced by coming out the other side of challenging experiences.

Servant leadership is steeped in humility. As mentioned, the distinction between equity leadership and servant leadership is that there is no intentionality about the impact of racialized oppression, identity oppression, or othering in the latter. We are all products of our environments and not naturally socialized to think about equity. We were raised in models that were/are "color blind." You might think that color doesn't make a difference. Perhaps you *don't see color*. Maybe when you see a Black person, you tell yourself you don't see a Black person. You just see a person … This is often the most offhanded and frustrating "compliment" (if you don't believe me, ask a colleague, friend, or confidant who is Black).

How do you give yourself permission in this era of tension to see the completeness of who we fully are in all our identities? There is no easy way around the *racialization* of that completeness. The *gendered* presence of that completeness. The *class* and *resource* lens of that completeness. These things just *are*. Equity leadership is groundbreaking and fundamental because it will not allow you to treat everyone the same. We're not all the same, and we don't all need the same things. As a leader, if you are striving or, dare I say, wanting to treat everyone the same, you're checking a box. This work requires a heavy dose of humility to see and acknowledge where other people are coming from. That is thinking differently …

This process requires unlearning certain messages and paradigms. There might be some collective principles I can apply to my team, but when I implement them individually, it will look very different from, say, Amy's experience or Nate's experience. *We must meet people at the point of their needs to meet the collective needs.* Giving everyone room at the table transforms challenges into *opportunities*. Something amazing happens when you lean into the word *opportunity* instead of *responsibility*.

> **WE MUST MEET PEOPLE AT THE POINT OF THEIR NEEDS TO MEET THE COLLECTIVE NEEDS.**

responsibility:

the state or fact of having a duty to deal with something or of having control over someone.

opportunity:

a set of circumstances that makes it possible to do something.

WHAT'S IN A WORD?

Names, once they are in common use, quickly become mere sounds, their etymology being buried, like so many of the earth's marvels, beneath the dust of habit.

—SALMAN RUSHDIE

Thinking differently requires analyzing words. For example, a commonly used definition of health equity is "the assurance of conditions for optimal health. For all people, achieving health equity requires valuing all individuals, all populations, *equally* recognizing and rectifying historical injustices, and providing resources."[3]

There is that conundrum of a word *equal*, and its synonym *same*. One of the biggest mixed messages in this society comes from defining fairness as *sameness*. "I treat all my patients/students/neighbors … the same." I would submit that one of the most unfair things we can do is to treat people the same. Sameness is not fairness. Figuring out the unique needs of individuals and populations must be *combined* with collective needs. We're deconstructing this assumption in a social hierarchy where white people are seen as better, Black men are seen as better than Black women, Christians are seen as better than Muslims,

---

3   "What Is Health Equity?" American Medical Association, July 17, 2022, https://www. ama-assn.org/delivering-care/health-equity/what-health-equity.

etc. Ironically, the concept of *equality* gets in the way of valuing the difference and uniqueness of who we are. We might do enough work as a society to one day apply *equality* for the best interests of all, but we're not there …

I'm not the same as you. I have three Black sons who aren't the same as your sons (even if they are Black). As a matter of fact, our hunger for sameness can be placated in the following diagram. In many ways we're alike; in other ways, we're like *some*; but in some ways, we're like *no other*. We are all uniquely, wonderfully, and lovingly made.

DIVERSITY AS A BRIDGE TO UNITY

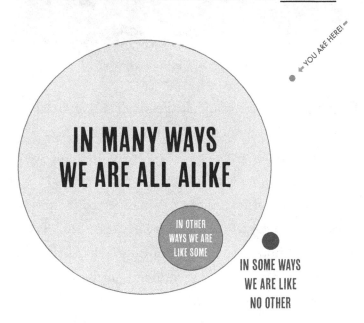

In the semantics of *equality*, there is little space for uniqueness. Equality wants us to all be right in the center, which is a lost opportunity. My family is richer because of the distinct personalities of three men who each check the box as "Renée's son." While they all check that same box, one is hilarious, one is musical, and one is compassionate. We need *all* that personality to make our family the best whole that it can be.

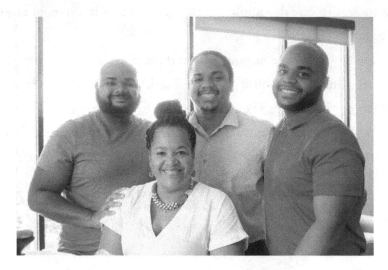

My sons, Marcus, Wesley, and Alexander

The Diversity, Equity, and Inclusion (DEI) professionals who are now employed in numerous organizations are likely wed to the term *inclusion*. But allow me to channel my third-grade teacher, Mr. Cook, who taught us *not to use a word to define itself*. Case in point— inclusion is the act of including. An unexpected definition of the word *include* is "to contain as a subordinate element." Perhaps it is the subtle implication of subordination (sounds like hierarchy to me) that impedes our effectiveness at authentic inclusion. In that case, inclusion is not the goal at all …

Another case in point: the common definition of the word *involvement* is also circular. "The fact or condition of being involved with or participating in something." Involvement is the condition of being involved. But if we look more closely at the definition of *involve*, we find it is "to include as a necessary circumstance or condition." How often do our efforts to include people make them feel just …

necessary, rather than welcome and vitally important? It is an echo of the term *tolerance*. (Who wants to be simply tolerated?)

This tension leads me to push us to think differently about another common phrase: *evidence-based practice*. All too often this term subordinates practice beneath evidence. In application, it is the subordination of community/practitioners beneath researchers/evidence producers. Why don't we talk more about *practice-based evidence*? It's an important distinction. The tension between these two phrases forces us to ask who gets to legitimize *knowing*. It's a discussion about power. *Who* is included and who is involved? And why?

As leaders, supposedly sitting where the "buck stops," we are also very good at parsing things out—illuminating dichotomies. I was trained as a quantitative researcher in graduate school when quantitative methodology was more highly valued because of its focus on numbers and analytics. We were softly socialized to see *qualitative* research as less than because it was not based in hard numbers and calculations; an oddly ironic opinion coming from a social science field that is looked upon as "soft" science by those described as bench researchers. The truth is that qualitative knowledge is in some ways more telling and more descriptive than quantitative data. But there is this looming question of how we, as a society, legitimize some ways of knowing and delegitimize others.

All too often, the idea of evidence-based practice fosters thoughts like "Here we are, the creators of the evidence, the researchers and the scientists, and here are all the things we've learned. Community—or whoever you are—you can use this to make what you do better. You can put this into practice!" If your initial reaction is "I don't do that, Renée!" challenge yourself to think about what you are unintentionally doing that contributes to this impression.

Qualitative data is as vital, informative, legitimate, and affirming as the other. Luckily for me, I can critique both these methods, having lived in both worlds. I worked for sixteen years as a member of the academy—a full-time professor and researcher—so my career has been a half-and-half approach to these research methodologies. I understand data collection and *other* ways of knowing. At the beginning of my academic career, the idea of being an applied sociologist was not highly regarded; it was about being a scholar and intellectual. Ways of knowing are diverse, so who gets to legitimize that? Ideally, concepts like evidence-based practice and practice-based evidence will bring researchers into the community, and conversely, invite the community into research in ways that involve them without subordination. We have work to do, and it will take equity leadership to get us there.

Fortunately, this is already happening. There are good examples of it … and terrible ones. Some partner with the community in ways that allow them to *check that box* and say, "I worked with the community. Let's just call it community-based or participatory research." Others truly come in with humility—with the soul of authentic equity and inclusion—and ask community partners, "What is a pressing problem or need that you have?" allowing them to set the research agenda and use their skills to help the community articulate and define a solution.

What is your authenticity litmus test? How are you checking and affirming that (1) you're being true to community participation as a leader, and (2) you're not slipping back into old habits? Are you being *vigilant?* As an equity leader, you must constantly monitor yourself for this! We're all socialized to see leadership as hierarchical. Resist the urge to lean back into old paradigms.

So much of this journey for me has been about unmasking leadership-based internalized oppression where you buy into negative constructs. We must work with intention. There's no space for old paradigms. None of this: *I'll just get it over with. It'll be better and faster this way.* Simply getting it done *might* be faster, but not better or more lasting. Your job is not to fix problems; your job is to create a culture that allows for reflection to collaboratively offer solutions and help implement those solutions.

Before sitting down to work on this chapter, I had a meeting with colleagues about updating and revising a graduate course. In attendance were academics and practitioners. Despite the diversity of backgrounds, the discussion was still pretty scholarly. Someone said, "I don't mean for this to be *polemic*, but—" They went on to their points, and I couldn't help but think to myself, *There's no local public health practitioner who is sitting in a conference room with colleagues discussing what seems* polemic*!* Don't get me wrong, it's a lovely word, and as I said before, I love words. My point is this: we often spend more time acting smart than *being* smart. We *act* like a leader rather than *leadering.* We seem oblivious to whom we're talking to—in other words, read the room! So maybe we just need more folx at the table. But let's take a moment to think about that word.

> **polemic:**
> *a strong verbal or written attack on someone or something.*

Perhaps not a bad word for us as equity leaders to be familiar with. Certainly, resistance and even verbal or written attacks often accompany our attempts to shift thinking. How do we prepare for the polemic? As well as for the disingenuousness of saying, "I don't mean to be polemic but …" and proceeding to be polemic! Or "I don't mean to be rude but …" and proceeding to be rude. "I'm not trying to offend anyone but …" and proceeding to offend. You get the point.

THINKING DIFFERENTLY TO SEE, SAY, AND DO DIFFERENTLY

*Prayer will help you think differently, view things
differently and do things differently.*

—GIFT GUGU MONA

This last section is a primer of sorts. Thinking differently is the gateway to *seeing, saying,* and *doing* differently. I'll give an example. I was serving on my local American Red Cross board of directors when the National Office released a pool safety poster. The title was "Be Cool, Follow the Rules." This poster had little white, Black, and Brown kids jumping into and playing around the pool. Their behavior was labeled (with an arrow) as either "cool" or "not cool." I had to laugh before I cried. Problematically, all the Black and Brown kids were exhibiting "not cool" behavior while the white kids were labeled as "cool"!

I would hazard a guess that there are plenty of white people who would never see that until they were told about it (especially those who *do not see color*). They didn't see it and then … they saw it, like my Chevy Cavalier story. Imagine the person on the design team who sat in a conference room and shared this *great* poster. Was the racial behavior delineation a part of their big plan? Who would have done that intentionally? The truth is, probably nobody. *Nobody* did that intentionally, I would hope. They just couldn't see it. This type of pattern has been replicated in numerous places and spaces—it is why there is so much present attention on implicit bias.[4] As an aside, the Red Cross was extremely responsive to the feedback and pulled the poster, but if there is any good from the implicit bias error, many have been helped to see differently as a result.

---

4   "Implicit Bias," American Psychological Association, accessed May 19, 2023, https://www.apa.org/topics/implicit-bias.

> **implicit bias:**
>
> *implicit bias, also known as implicit prejudice or implicit attitude, is a negative attitude, of which one is not consciously aware, against a specific social group.*

As you begin to think and see differently, you position yourself to give voice to different mental models and worldviews—saying differently … We become more mindful of the words we choose. This is not political correctness. Political correctness is about conforming. *Saying differently* in the context of equity leadership is about transforming. We are mindful of words and phrases that offend or exclude because authentic relationships require us to do so. Our goal is to transform our agencies, communities, cities, regions, and other spaces of influence in ways that can honor the depth of relationships—keeping people whole and at the table. If you know someone well, you not only know what is offensive but also *why* it is offensive. The choice to avoid saying things that damage relationships is just that—a choice that is willingly made.

I often say that equity leadership can't be taught but it can be *learned*. That may seem existential, but I can stand up front for twenty hours lecturing till I'm blue in the face or write twenty books to be read, but until you choose to engage, you will not learn and behavior will not change. *You have to unlearn before you can learn. You dig into and disrupt long-held assumptions to make space for foundational content for equity leadership.* For example, you have to

YOU HAVE TO UNLEARN BEFORE YOU CAN LEARN. YOU DIG INTO AND DISRUPT LONG-HELD ASSUMPTIONS TO MAKE SPACE FOR FOUNDATIONAL CONTENT FOR EQUITY LEADERSHIP.

unlearn the principle that race doesn't matter, that we should all be color blind, or that the United States is a melting pot.

Choose to unlearn these principles so that you can teach this reality of the social construction of race and how it influences people's lives. You're already *thinking differently*, and then, and only then, can you learn for *yourself*. I'm not standing in front of you right now proclaiming, "Here I am! Presenting to you, the light bulb moment! Here's a new idea, the 'aha.' I'm the educator, trainer, and workshop facilitator. Thou shalt now be an equity titan!"

It should be easy to teach these concepts, but, if we stick with the light bulb analogy, some people simply have no sockets to screw in that bulb. Many individuals are closed to new ideas. I have no holder for this bright idea that I'm endeavoring to teach if someone chooses not to learn. There is a dialectic back and forth between a teacher and learner, tutor and professor, mentor and mentee, or coach and athlete. There's got to be a *willingness*.

How do you, future equity leader, get to that place of "Yep, I'm going to allow myself to think differently about this so that I can start *seeing* differently, *saying* differently, and, ultimately, *doing* differently?" If you still don't know, there's no need to worry. Let's delve deeper into seeing differently.

LEARNING LESSONS: THINKING DIFFERENTLY

- You don't have to do this work; you *get* to do this work ...
- Humility is the equity container for holding space with others.
- Meet people at the place of their needs. We're not equal!
- Thinking differently is the gateway to *seeing*, *saying*, and *doing* differently.

MIRROR MOMENTS: THINKING DIFFERENTLY

1. Think of a time when you "studied long and studied wrong" (i.e., you thought you were right about a fact but realized you were completely wrong). How did you move toward understanding and accepting the different/correct frame?
2. What does it usually take for you to change your mind about a position? How are you best persuaded in those cases (facts, feelings, experiences, etc.)?
3. Reflect on a paradigm that you were taught as a child that you no longer hold as an adult. How did this shift change your way of operating in the world?

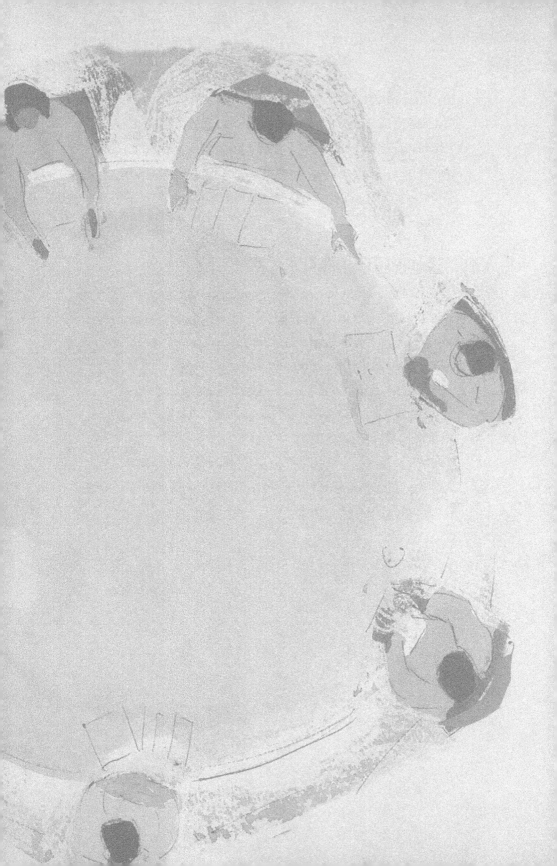

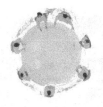

CHAPTER FOUR

MAKING THE INVISIBLE VISIBLE

That invisibility to which I refer occurs because of a peculiar disposition of the eyes of those with whom I come in contact. A matter of the construction of their INNER eyes, those eyes with which they look through their physical eyes upon reality.

— RALPH ELLISON

H ave you ever been directed by someone to look in a particular direction to see something that *they* see and you simply cannot see? Perhaps you were at a concert or graduation and your friend said, "There's John," pointing with clarity in a certain direction. The conversation continues with you saying, "I don't see him." Your friend replies, "He's right there!" pointing more emphatically. It goes on like this: "I don't see him." "He's right there, you can't miss him!" "Where?!" "Right there!" etc., and just before the two of you implode into a puddle of frustration, you exclaim, "Oh, right there! I *see* him now …" What happened at that moment when the invisible became visible?

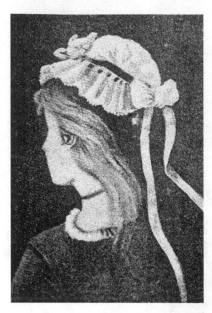

"Seeing Differently"

Sometimes it's a bit more inexplicable. Consider the optical illusion above. The question surrounding the image is "What do you see in this picture?" You might see a young woman or you may see an old woman in this illusion known as "My mother in law and my wife." Which do you see? More importantly, how is it that we can look at the same image and see completely different things? Your context, in this case your age and experience or comfort with aging, shape what you see.

Hans Christian Andersen wrote "The Emperor's New Clothes" in 1837. This fictitious tale is about a monarch obsessed with his apparel—consumed to the point that he's conned by "weavers" who promise him fabric so light that it's invisible to those who are ... well ... considered stupid. This leads the arrogant emperor to show off his new outfit—ultimately, he's in his birthday suit—to his subjects, who give him thunderous applause and enthusiastically congratulate him. Conversely, we convince ourselves to (pretend to) see things that simply *are not* there. In a society where racism exists but we tell ourselves the opposite—falling into groupthink or social hysteria—we agree that *what we know deep down is not the case.* It's buried.

I am not a neuropsychologist and couldn't begin to provide physiological or clinical explanations for what is occurring. But I am a sociologist and see the implications of how we are socialized to see and interpret the world around us. How do people's backgrounds affect how they *see?* When you're socialized to view the world in a certain way, it's hard to unlearn. I'll keep telling you: we see things not as *they* are but as *we* are. The young lad who spoke up at the end of "The Emperor's New Clothes" provides equity leaders with a great question. *Will we be the brave soul who speaks up, even when others try to silence us?*

> WILL WE BE THE BRAVE SOUL WHO SPEAKS UP, EVEN WHEN OTHERS TRY TO SILENCE US?

It is hard to deny that we live in a society crippled by our history of racism, sexism, ableism, and other -isms. But when those around us keep shaking their heads in denial, thinking, "No such thing!" we who are social justice advocates must step in and sound the alarm. "The emperor has no clothes!" *Hello!* "Will we all pretend that he *isn't* in the nude?"

Society inclines us to reprimand the seers. "Don't say that about our glorious emperor, kid! Don't say it because you will completely disrupt our worldview and mental models." And as equity leaders, this is precisely our goal! We can no longer ignore or refuse to see the racialized patterns all around us. I have heard the question "Why is everything about race for you all?" Well, how is it not about race for so many? *The emperor has no clothes!*

People continue to ask why we're still talking about racism. Many want to stop seeing issues that make them uncomfortable. I would offer that recent executive orders at the federal, state, and county levels that pushed to ban contractors from providing "racial sensitivity training" are an extreme effort to keep people from seeing differently. The arguments that such trainings "indoctrinate government employees with divisive and harmful sex and race-based ideologies" is simply erroneous. I argue that is a Rorschach spot reaction - their interpretation is reflected more by their worldview than by what the present, see-able reality for many. All too often, society desperately wishes to keep its eyes shut.

> I HAVE HEARD THE QUESTION "WHY IS EVERYTHING ABOUT RACE FOR YOU ALL?" WELL, HOW IS IT NOT ABOUT RACE FOR SO MANY?

FREEDOM IN SEEING

Open my eyes, that I may behold wondrous things out of your law.

—PSALM 119:18

There is freedom in seeing. Racial healing begins with seeing. You can't resolve the pain until you allow yourself to see the pain. We attain collective victory when we collectively realize that we're not winning. Someone who can't see it might ask, "What do you mean we're not winning?" Well, we aren't ... There is a narrative of patriotism in this country that blinds us to myths and flaws that keep many issues invisible. This flawed narrative seems to suggest that if we see the need for growth, improvement, and change in our country, then we lack patriotism. As you'll recall, nothing could be further from the truth.

Equity work is the opposite of antipatriotism. I am an equity leader who believes in this country and the ideals of what it can be.

There are numerous things that keep us from seeing, including things like no awareness of the reality of oppression, consciously protecting one's own privilege, guilt or shame, fear of being cast as the oppressor, the culture of politeness, media reinforcement of stereotypes, collective values such as individualism and meritocracy, and so much more. Personally deconstructing the impact of any one of these would help bring clarity and sight.

Unfortunately, equity leadership is still groundbreaking. It asks you to open your eyes and stop peeping through apprehensive fingers to avoid seeing the whole picture. One of the characteristics needed to open your eyes is curiosity (also translated as the twin of nosiness by some!). Is it possible that you may be missing something? Are you curious enough to take what might seem like a risk and peek? Engender in yourself that willingness to say—to recognize—that there are some things we may not see, especially without the help of others.

The quote above from the book of Psalms is a request for help, assistance in seeing more clearly. Seeing is sometimes a partnered event, developed from relationship with others who have different perspectives. Increasing comfort with discomfort is one of the common agreements in health equity and social justice work. No one innately wants to be uncomfortable. As soon as we get uncomfortable, it seems like the fight-or-flight response kicks in, and we want to run away. But I can assure you that the discomfort is fleeting. It does not last forever. And consequently, your lens seems much broader because you were willing to be uncomfortable.

I do love the blue jeans metaphor. After comfortably wearing those jeans several times, you throw them in the wash. Somehow, when you put the clean jeans back on, they are uncomfortable! They require more tug and pull to get them on. Well, the longer you wear them, the more comfortable they get. The same goes for equity. The longer you have these discussions about the issues that divide us—like race and racism—the more comfortable you become having these conversations. You cross a point, and the comfort returns.

We don't seem to trust that comfort will return. But somehow it does. The discomfort dampens. It's now easier for me to discuss race, oppression, and gender discrimination because I've had *so many* conversations along these lines. Are they one hundred percent comfortable, even for me? Absolutely not! Note that I said they are *easier* and I did not say they are *easy*. But I've had enough experience to trust that it will get comfortable as I persevere, and I persevere because building relationship across difference is vital to creating change.

For another example, think about the experience of getting in the pool. People who are already in the pool tell you to "Get in. It's really warm. It feels great!" So you put your foot in the water and think to yourself, *This is not warm. It's cold! I'm not getting in.* Then you somehow coax yourself into the pool. After a few minutes of discomfort, you're swimming and splashing, giving no thought to the temperature of the water, except perhaps a brief reflection on how strange it was that you thought the water was frigid at the beginning. The benefits of engaging in potentially difficult discussions, like floating in that wonderful pool, far outweigh the consequences of not engaging or not diving in!

REMOVING THE BLINDERS

We must reinvent a future free of blinders so that we can choose from real options.

—DAVID SUZUKI

Many wonder how we get people to approach this work if they're stubborn or stuck in their privilege or blindness. Recognizing that stuck things can become unstuck is an important start. In many ways, color blindness is a manifestation of privilege blindness. The underlying goal of blindness in the battle for this work is the preference for not seeing—for keeping the invisible unseen.

Peggy McIntosh famously authored the article entitled "Unpacking the Invisible Knapsack." Using pragmatic examples, it makes the earlier point that protecting privilege or no awareness of privilege often keeps us from seeing oppression. The most erroneous part of that orientation is the oft-unspoken assumption that this work is about *taking away* privilege or power … It is not. Heather McGhee's book, *The Sum of Us: What Racism Costs Everyone and How We Can Prosper Together*, hits the nail on the head with her explanation of the principle of *one-sum gain*—if *you* gain something, that does not mean *I* have lost something. This work is not about loss. It is about the benefit for us all.

I'M NOT MORE POWERFUL BECAUSE I IGNORE YOUR POWER. I'M MORE POWERFUL WHEN I SEE AND POSITION YOU TO EMBRACE YOUR POWER. AS INDIVIDUALS, WE CAN BE STRATEGIC ABOUT OUR POWER, AND ALIGNING OUR POWER FOR COLLECTIVE INFLUENCE IS AN EFFECTIVE STRATEGY FOR CHANGE.

I'm not a fan of the aphorisms "a rising tide lifts all boats" or "leveling the playing field," but what I glean from them is that just because my boat is rising, it doesn't mean yours is sinking. It is a myth that if you gain power, I lose power. Similarly, leveling the field allows for no variation based on needs, preferences, or priorities and discounts the fact that we do not all need the same thing. The truth is that we *all* have power, some recognized and some unrecognized.

Again, a call to pull down the veil or go behind the curtain and make the unseen seen—the invisible visible.

We have *different levels of influence*. I'm not more powerful because I ignore your power. I'm more powerful when I see and position you to embrace your power. As individuals, we can be strategic about our power, and aligning our power for collective influence is an effective strategy for change. Consider something as simple as your possessing this book (owned or borrowed!). The very fact that you have the resources to purchase *Room at the Table*, or the *relationship* resources from somebody who gifted or loaned you this book, demonstrates power or privilege in a very fundamental way. You are actively seeking to expand your capacity to embrace your power as you pursue the goal of equity leadership …

The freedom and willingness to *see* begins with yourself—understanding that your worldview and mindset are critical in *shaping* what you see, how you see it, or how you overlook it. Recognizing how to unlearn myths and mindsets is needed to make room for new and more applicable equity frames, no matter your sphere of influence. It's ironic because I describe myself as others focused. I receive the greatest gratification when I help you achieve your goals. But the only reason I can focus on you is that I have previously focused on myself (and continue to do so). I have figured out my "stuff" that could potentially get in the way of an authentic and effective lens for seeing inequities—inequities that impede equity leadership and, as a result, create barriers to authentic relationship.

The absence of self-awareness is another significant weakness of an equity leader. All too often we get in our own way. When considering personal and interpersonal domains, there is no getting around ourselves as the potential source of the problem but also as a potential solution to the problem. Your Mirror Moments are opportunities to learn about yourself ... We tend to avoid self-reflection out of fear that *we* are the source of the problem, but recognizing that we *might be* is actually beneficial! Perspective, position, priority. Understand that self-reflection is one of the first steps to being an equity leader. *See* your courageous self, in all its incarnations, tribulations, and viewpoints.

We put blinders on other creatures—literally and figuratively— to control what they see. As equity leaders, it is our responsibility to recognize if we are *wearing* blinders and who or what has placed them over our eyes. Systems, worldviews, and mental models often seek to blind and resist change. Social blinders keep us moving in the same old direction, avoiding much-needed change and growth in our society. Removing the blinders might make you and others vulnerable, and it may also instigate grappling, but we collectively heal by making the invisible visible. We set each other free. "Lean into the discomfort of the work," says Casandra Brené Brown. Yes, my friends. Let's courageously *see* ourselves and others.

ECOLOGICAL FALLACY

Ecological fallacy is a failure in reasoning that arises when an inference is made about an individual based on aggregate data for a group.

—BRITANNICA

When engaging in conversations about race and racism, I often hear the retort, "Well, I didn't own slaves. Why do I have to be blamed for all this?" First of all, *feeling* blamed and *being* blamed are two very different things. But even the mention of institutional racism can cause people to become defensive. They think you're calling them a racist. It compels me to want to sit down, have a one-on-one, and say, "Can I ask you a little bit more about that? What is it about a conversation on institutional racism that makes you feel it's personally about you?"

History is history, and none of us chose what race or gender we would be born into. No one chose their poverty level or, conversely, the wealth of the family into which they would be born. There is indeed personal and self-reflective work that needs to be done on this journey. To excessively internalize these issues gets in the way of racial healing as a society and personal growth as an equity leader. Yet, contrary to the "don't take this personally" comment, we need to take these matters personally in order to assess our role and change our actions.

Embarrassment, guilt, or shame do not fuel equity change. They have the opposite effect—getting in the way. So negative reactions to this work are triggers or hints that either we need to stay at the table (privilege can entice us to leave it) or we need to work to keep others at the table. This work is not calling anyone a racist—it allows racism to be visible so that we might collectively heal. But … *what keeps people out of the room and away from the table is a case of what I would describe as ecological fallacy.*

> **ecological fallacy:**
>
> *ecological fallacy, also called ecological inference fallacy in epidemiology, [is a] failure in reasoning that arises when an inference is made about an individual based on aggregate data for a group.*

Ecological fallacy highlights that any trend at the group level might erroneously be applied to the individual. Let's use a public health example and discuss smoking. Smoking cessation is an important public health goal, but from an epidemiological perspective, we need to see things differently. If we look at a collection of people with lung cancer, most of them had a smoking history. That doesn't mean I can look at you, an individual who *is* a smoker, and say, "You will get cancer." That is an ecological fallacy. Dare I say, not seeing the trees for the forest …

Ecological fallacy also shapes our mindsets and how we view race and racism. Institutionally, numerous patterns surround us that reveal *disproportionate disadvantages* for some groups over others. Still, that doesn't mean that you, Mr./Mrs./Miss Individual, are a racist. What we endeavor to make visible is institutional, structural racism. Ecological fallacy highlights thinking that is too broad and overgen-

> WHAT KEEPS PEOPLE OUT OF THE ROOM AND AWAY FROM THE TABLE IS A CASE OF WHAT I WOULD DESCRIBE AS ECOLOGICAL FALLACY.

eralized. It keeps alive the assumptions that allow the invisible to remain invisible—assumptions that make people run. They leave the table, not understanding the larger goal of equity leadership.

We are living through the consequences, impacts of decisions, and choices that far predated us. All the more reason to not live with blinders on. Many leaders are in a comfortable place, tempted to say, "It's not affecting *me*." Good enough isn't good enough! Because you have this book in your hands, you're not in the "I don't see color," "don't talk about it," and "let's leave things alone" category. You're putting on those freshly washed blue jeans and finding a way to compel others to do the same. When ecological fallacy takes people away from the table, you extend your hand and invite them back.

THE CULTURE OF POLITENESS—STOP SEEING!

Politeness is organized indifference.

—PAUL VALÉRY

Structured racism parades behind social norms—people with good manners don't talk about money, income, religion, etc. Part of our job is to play the forensic detective. We have to challenge ourselves and ask, "When did we decide it was rude to talk with someone about how much money they make, how they identify racially, what, if any, religion they follow, and why?" When did we decide this was business as usual? How did the public narrative get established as such? In our social norms, not wanting to talk about these things was inculcated into the ethos of this nation, and not only did these topics become taboo, but they also set the tone for *if we didn't say it, then we didn't see it.*

THE CULTURE OF POLITENESS IS REINFORCED IN THAT FIRST EXPERIENCE OF PUTTING A FOOT IN OUR MOUTH, AND THEN WE KNOW NOT TO REPEAT THE OFFENSE. THIS LEARNING SETS A COLLECTIVE TONE OF CAUTIOUSNESS THAT PUSHES US TO SEE NOTHING.

We are socialized into this public narrative as children when we make comments like "That lady's dress is old and dirty!" or "Why don't you go to church!" The parent's reprimand of *shh* begins our training into discomfort. In some ways, we're taught to be inauthentic. Alas, therein lies the culture of politeness. *The culture of politeness is reinforced in that first experience of putting a foot in our mouth, and then we know not to repeat the offense. This learning sets a collective tone of cautiousness that pushes us to see nothing.* "I shouldn't see it," in action, translates to "I just won't say anything." Being extremely cautious turns into silence. "I don't see it! It's better to say nothing. It's better to be disingenuous and silent than to say something and risk offending." But even being the source of an offense elevates the opportunity to push toward authentic relationship.

When we are taught to be silent in response to sensitive matters, we are essentially trained not to see other vitally important topics. These deeply ingrained lessons require unlearning. Unpacking our silence, and that of others, is a way to unlearn and understand the silence response. Equity leadership encourages people to see and speak—especially through discomfort. If something comes out wrong, it becomes a learning opportunity, and at least you saw something and said something!

MONEY AND MERITOCRACY—SEEING DEEPER

Not everything that is profitable is of social value and
not everything of social value is profitable.

—JOHN T. HARVEY

Some colleagues and I recently went on a business-development trip to connect with existing and potential clients. We met with a leader at a large for-profit consulting firm, the culture of which is pretty distinct from ours as a smaller nonprofit firm. It happened that we were all African American leaders in this meeting, a somewhat rare occurrence. While that may have been a unifying factor, the potential partner's perspective was "Let me be clear, I'm a capitalist, and so how is your approach going to make money?" That was the undertone of the entire conversation. This person had clearly shaken off the culture of politeness! His priority, which started with the economic end in mind, seemed drawn from this conclusion that *social* good will cost money or not make money. Well, it may also save money or even generate money. And it very well may result in other benefits.

Making the invisible visible occurs when strongly held narratives are disrupted often through our openness to alternate points of view. Two strong examples are the *New York Times* article by Tamara C. Belinfanti titled, "Social Good Is Not Inconsistent with Profit," and the John T. Harvey *Forbes* article "Why Government Should Not Be Run like a Business." Harvey summarizes the problem: "Not everything that is profitable is of social value and not everything of social value is profitable." We're talking apples and oranges. There's a dichotomy here.

The potential partner, after informing me that he is a *capitalist*, wanted to make sure we'd make money. All right. One business's "making money" is another business's breaking even. So many economic metrics require comparison; wealth and poverty are relative. The costs of not addressing equity as leaders may not be directly financial, but there are costs to turning a blind eye. There are things we choose to do as a society simply because it's the right thing to do. We might not make money off them, but they *will* profit us. The public narrative that questions what is more important, health or money, can be circular. Social good can be measured in numerous ways other than money. Equity leadership requires reconciling a narrative of opposites.

The issue of revenue propels me to consider the concept of meritocracy, which assumes that some people or ventures are more worthwhile or of greater worth than others. The idea of *pulling yourself up by your bootstraps* is just flawed thinking, in my opinion, but it is so deeply rooted in our social narrative in the United States. Pulling yourself up by your bootstraps, in many ways, is an ecological fallacy—assuming that a group of highly successful people worked hard, so if all individuals worked hard, they would also succeed. I know many frustrated hardworking people who have not experienced the *fruit* of their efforts.

I'll turn to my beloved sons as an example. They're in their midtwenties and early thirties. Recently, they shared the story of a friend whose parents gave them a house as a wedding gift. I had to reflect on that for a moment. I have a good job, and I'm blessed with a wonderful salary, but I teasingly said to my sons, "You know I work hard but I can't give y'all a house!" The parents who gifted that home didn't necessarily have self-earned wealth, but *their* parents had given them similarly substantive gifts—that is what generational wealth looks like; it is often bootstrap-free!

Generational wealth is a wonderful thing, but it is not as simple as *I worked so hard, and now I have these bootstraps. I'm a self-made person.* Somehow, people who ascribe to that narrative don't see the generational setup that benefited them. The absence of college or housing debt, and the availability of discretionary income through trust funds—multiple streams of income are not benefits that are ascribed to all, despite our claim to be the land of opportunity. In many cases, it's not about what you did but what you *didn't have to do*. Most communities of color aren't in that position.

For centuries, African American families weren't using the revenue and income they generated to store up and save for the future. What they earned as enslaved people went to slave owners. It's not that we didn't work hard. The stereotype that Blacks are lazy is beyond ironic. This point makes it all the more *incredible* that we're positioned on the crux of making the invisible visible. The concept of social privilege—especially racial privilege—is very challenging for many, particularly white Americans who grew up in situations of poverty and lack (by the way, this is another occasion of ecological fallacy).

It's hard for many white Americans to see how their lineage might have positioned them to exist in a system that was structured for their benefit. It is easier to assume that they worked hard in college and got a good job. These are "both/and" conditions—hard work paired with historical benefit, even if unseen. It is also a challenge to measure what *didn't* happen—the bias and stereotyping that did *not* occur. A reverse example: the résumé that was overlooked because of the ethnic-appearing name.

Numerous systems operate in seemingly invisible ways, without a large contingent of those who want to bring the inequitable actions to light. It's as though we refuse to see them. Imagine a toddler playing hide and seek who covers their eyes and cries out with glee, "You can't see me!" We actually do see you, but will go along with the ruse. You don't see it till you see it, and are you willing to act on what you see? Many Black, Brown, and Indigenous people are working hard, and white Americans who don't have the benefit of generational wealth are doing the same. But when we look at the big picture, white Americans are vastly more likely to possess inherited wealth than Black Americans. We also know that the consequences of this pattern reach far beyond bank accounts—wealth is also health and well-being.

As a maternal child health researcher, I saw consistent findings that Black women with college degrees are still more likely to experience higher infant mortality rates than white women who haven't finished high school.[5] So when controlling for education and economics, that unexplained variance seemed to allude to the experiences and consequences of racism. These empirical findings were also my own lived

---

5   Samuel H. Fishman et al., "Race/Ethnicity, Maternal Educational Attainment, and Infant Mortality in the United States," *Biodemography and Social Biology* 66, no. 1 (January–March 2020): 1–26, doi:10.1080/19485565.2020.1793659.

experience as a college-educated Black woman whose firstborn son was delivered at twenty-eight weeks and lost his life at six months due to complications of prematurity and RSV.

"Land of the free, home of the brave." This remarkable country simply isn't the land of opportunity for everyone. I would submit that when leaders, through a committed equity lens, begin to deconstruct some of these illusions, then and only then can we rebuild systems that will indeed do what we say and ultimately broaden advantage. We can love our country while still seeing, inviting others to see, and then taking the next step ... *saying* something.

LEARNING LESSONS: MAKING THE INVISIBLE VISIBLE

- You don't see it till you see it.
- Try the jeans on again—discomfort leads to comfort.
- The culture of politeness leads to the culture of blindness.
- Look past the ROI models—equity work doesn't need to be profitable to be beneficial.

MIRROR MOMENTS: MAKING THE INVISIBLE VISIBLE

1. Recall an aha moment, and describe a figurative or actual time when you didn't see something until you saw it (like the optical illusion).
2. What assumptions have you placed upon others because of ecological fallacy?
3. Reflect on your heritage. What generational challenges or advantages have contributed to your being where you are today?

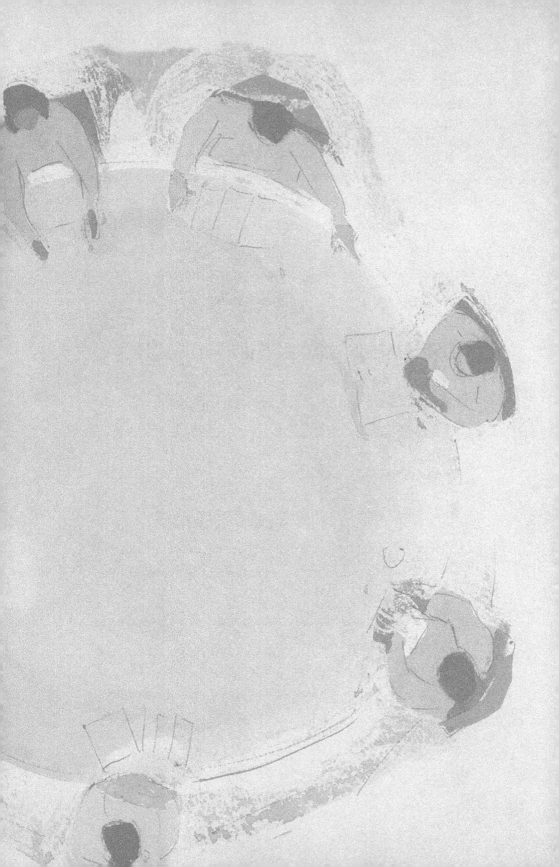

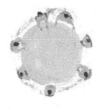

CHAPTER FIVE

AUTHENTIC COMMUNICATION

You own everything that happened to you. Tell your stories. If people wanted you to write warmly about them, they should've behaved better.

— ANNE LAMOTT

My grandmother used to say, "Everybody grinnin' ain't tickled, and everybody crying ain't sad." Now I want you to reread that quote and hear it with a sweet southern drawl underscoring that point and prodding the hearer to think deeply about the words she was sharing. Her quote speaks to authenticity and naivete. Similarly, I would offer the colloquialism that "everybody sayin' equity don't mean equity." In other words, we can no longer naively assume that everyone saying *health equity* authentically means health equity. What is really lurking behind that grin or that word?

There seems to be some level of social pressure. All the "cool kids" are saying health equity, so you probably should also say it! That is the worst-case scenario. Even the best case may only be that they *understand* what it means but don't know what to *do* about it. There are two forms of opposition posing significant threats to our advancing equity: (1) There are those saying equity to shut us up. "If I say this enough (health equity), maybe it'll go away …" and (2) there are those refusing to say equity and seeking strategies to force us not to say it. We have even seen executive orders at the federal level and proposed laws at the state level. When has censorship ever been a rational strategy!

As equity leaders, we must be discerning. Hearing someone use the term *equity* is not in and of itself sufficient. It would be easy to slide into a space of comfort, or even complacency, and convince ourselves that we can move forward because someone has added the word *equity* to their conversation. How do we assess someone's commitment and authenticity based upon what they say?—observing their reactions and responses to challenging dialogue and *challenges in dialogue*. What indicators of authenticity do you observe?

It is often difficult to interpret the true intent of others when we're doing this work. People can be disingenuous, but we also may be misinterpreting their words or reactions, as implied by the second part of my grandmother's quote: "everybody crying ain't sad." Silence, laughter, tears, and other expressions can have multiple meanings. "She's crying. Give her a tissue. Don't cry." But maybe she's not crying because she's sad. Perhaps she's crying because she was deeply moved by something or crying because she's happy to finally see a glimmer of hope. And perhaps the flowing tears are a cathartic representation that shouldn't simply be wiped away. We must strive to accurately interpret the motives behind people's actions or expressions. Authentic communication is birthed from authentic relationship.

INTENT VERSUS IMPACT

intent:

motive or purpose.

impact:

to have an effect on; influence; alter.

I was once a guest panelist for the American Medical Association Center for Health Equity during the COVID-19 pandemic, and as a point of dialogue, the host showed a picture of a billboard with an adorable Black baby. The headline read, "I am an outbreak." This image was immediately nonsensical, and my internal conversation went something like this: *What did y'all think you were doing with this campaign—a baby of color with the phrase "I'm an outbreak"? What on earth?* Ultimately, it was shared that the intended message was to encourage parents to get their kids vaccinated.

Much like the American Red Cross poster mentioned previously, I wish I could have been a fly on the wall during the committee meeting that designed the billboard. I imagine that they did not discuss how to develop *the most offensive campaign possible.* The irony is that the campaign was likely more alienating of the population that they were seeking to draw in. Thankfully, the image resulted in a powerful panel discussion and case example at that moment—intent versus impact. What do we do when the consequences of our words or actions are unintentionally negative?

Imagine an incident where someone (or perhaps even you) accidentally says something offensive, especially in the context of exchanges across race. The reaction tends to be, "Well, I didn't mean it that way." But the unspoken undercurrent of that statement is often "and because

I didn't mean it that way, you shouldn't be offended." *But the words that came out of your mouth were offensive!* A common aphorism chastens that stance—"The road to hell is paved with good intentions." If I might take a bit of poetic license with the well-known quote from Peter Drucker, I'd argue that impact eats intent for breakfast! I'm not suggesting that intent is irrelevant, but when intent and impact work against each other, our responsibility as equity leaders is always to take responsibility for the impact of our actions.

TAKING RESPONSIBILITY COMES DOWN TO LEARNING WHY SOMETHING WAS OFFENSIVE AND FACILITATING HEALING AFTER HARM HAS BEEN CAUSED.

Taking responsibility comes down to learning why something was offensive and facilitating healing after harm has been caused. The place to begin is an authentic apology. It is interesting how often attempts to apologize end up contributing to more angst. One observation is the inclusion of the simple two-letter word *if*—this word never belongs in an authentic apology. Why not? For one, you know that you have offended, which is why you are endeavoring to apologize, and secondly, that posture appears to seek absolution of sorts, seemingly beckoning the response, "Oh, you didn't offend me." No, you know that you have offended them! That's why you're apologizing.

I offer an effective word replacement—"I'm sorry *that* I offended you," demonstrates the acceptance of responsibility as well as accountability for the impact of our actions. This statement forces you to take responsibility even when you may want the interaction to just go away. You didn't wish to harm or hurt anyone, but you did. I can recall numerous occasions when I ended up oddly comforting the person who caused my offense, and at my own expense.

What sets equity leaders apart is that we confront courageously—we process and think through challenges, not just blow them off with a simple word, statement, or lackluster apology. I'm sure you've heard the pushback before. Here are a few relationship-damaging, nonchalant rebuffs, masquerading as apologies:

- You know I didn't mean it that way.
- Oh, don't take things so seriously.
- You're overreacting.
- Here we go again.
- Well, you *know* what I meant.

No to all of these! The person who has been offended knows what they *felt*.

The recipient of the misguided words is already harmed. Avoiding the hurt of others that has been caused by our actions or words is a neglect of our responsibility. Leaders who apply an equity lens seek to understand their hand in the offense and cultivate a strategy for not having a similarly problematic engagement happen in the future. Equity leaders make space for their discomfort to engage in ways that allow growth and healing.

"UNCEASING" MIRROR MOMENTS

This above all: to thine own self be true,
And it must follow, as the night the day,
Thou canst not then be false to any man.

—WILLIAM SHAKESPEARE

I have found that my greatest strength—dare I say my superpower—as an equity-driven leader is vulnerability, honesty, and risk-taking.

The fuel that powers the operationalization of these strengths is *self-reflection*. For example, confessing that I am uncomfortable is one of the most effective prefaces in a difficult dialogue across difference (race, gender, etc.)

- This is really a hard conversation for me, but ...
- I'm going to lean into some discomfort and say ...
- I trust that I can be transparent with you ...
- I'm going to take a risk and say ...

Approaching a dialogue this way lowers *my* guard because, if they overreact, I can refer them back to my preface. I disclosed that it would be awkward, uncomfortable, etc. for me. This strategy has kept the space for dialogue open because those with whom I am engaging realize that they are not the only fish out of water in this exchange. It is mutual, and we are hopefully moving forward together. It is also effective because this is not an exclusively cognitive discourse. In this regard, I often frame such an encounter with the statement, "I hope you'll hear my heart and not my head." This is indeed head and heart work, both cognitive and affective.

> I'M TRYING TO GET YOU TO NOT JUST THINK COGNITIVELY, BUT ALSO AFFECTIVELY—THE MEANING, CONSEQUENCE, AND FEELING OF AN EVENT.

Affective. Yes, in equity work, there's much evidence at our fingertips. The facts are present. You can look at several statistics that reinforce challenges across race. But *I'm trying to get you to not just think cognitively, but also affectively—the meaning, consequence, and feeling of an event.* Asking someone to "Hear my heart on this," requires that I share my heart, and that can be risky. It also requires me to have my own Mirror Moment and assess my motive. Is it honorable, selfless, and genuine? What is my sincerity in any given situation? This is a different conversation than if I were throwing out facts—225 Black men were shot by police in 2022, etc.[6] That is all factual. Rather, I'm trying to get people to think about the heart of the matter instead of the more callous response that I have heard where one retorts, "Well, they shouldn't have been running from the police."

Introducing compassion as a necessary ingredient in engagement with those who are different from ourselves is vital. Could you, for a moment, think with me about why Black men might run from the police? What type of fear would drive someone to flee on foot when they've got a gun pointed at their back? Why would someone be willing to take on such tremendous odds—in their mind, they could possibly get away—when the likelihood is that they won't succeed? These are affective and statistical considerations. Looking deeper …

We are examining and grappling with complex issues to bring reconciliation, growth, and strength to our organizations, communities, nation, and selves. How do we bring an affective, compassionate, graceful perspective? This is not a "fake it till you make it" scenario; we need to be authentic when we approach these issues. We must be sincere, and ultimately the whole purpose of communication is to reach understanding and perhaps even reconciliation. There are those who cannot grasp any perspective other their own. Polarization is the antithesis of authentic communication. Authentic communication says, "I'm not here to convince you to think what I think. I'm here for us to sincerely understand each other—to listen and hold space together." And perhaps out of that, we find the ties that bind us.

I'll reference my favorite Shakespeare quote: "To thine own self be true." Pull out that hand mirror, look into your own eyes, and be

---

6   "Number of People Shot to Death by Police in the United States from 2017–2023, by Race," Statista, March 29, 2023, https://www.statista.com/statistics/585152/ people-shot-to-death-by-us-police-by-race/.

true to yourself so that you can be authentic with others. I love the ease of Shakespeare's writing in this famous passage. I know that I don't have to be perfect, but if I'm true to myself, then as the night follows the day ... *Authentic communication is facilitated when we know ourselves and take time to reflect.* There's no effort that we must personally invest for the night to follow the day; it just does. Similarly, the process of authentic communication comes naturally when you are, first and foremost, yourself.

I think Shakespeare hit the nail on the head. When you are true to yourself, you'll be true to others. You won't tiptoe around difficult subjects. Again, vigilance is calling upon us. I love the arts, so I'll share another analogy. Take off your pointe shoes. This is not toe shoe ballet. We want your flat-footed truth in this situation. When we choose to be vulnerable, to be true to ourselves, we have the grounding and strength that allows us to make space for the vulnerability of others.

AUTHENTIC COMMUNICATION IS FACILITATED WHEN WE KNOW OURSELVES AND TAKE TIME TO REFLECT.

I am still working to be consistent in this regard. My journey remains in process. Leadership is as much a journey—if not more so—than a destination. Most of us are in leadership positions because we have had a series of progressively increasing responsibilities and successes, leading to a position that affords groundbreaking accomplishment. For equity leaders, it is not about the position but rather the positioning (*leadering*). We have been positioned to advance change in systems and people. This awakens in others the desire to receive our authentic communication. But always keep in mind the reverse! Can you, as an equity leader, receive authentic communication from another when it doesn't necessarily reconcile with yourself?

Authentic communication is bidirectional, as are intent and impact. Approach every difficult dialogue after you have your Mirror Moment. Know where you stand.

CULTURAL COMPETENCE AS A STRATEGY

The term cultural competence *describes a set of skills, values, and principles that acknowledge, respect, and contribute to effective interactions between individuals and the various cultural and ethnic groups they come in contact with at work and in their personal lives.*

— HUMANSERVICESEDU.ORG

The above is useful even if convoluted, but I've never found a more salient and simple definition of cultural competence than that by the social worker James Green. He defined cultural competence as the ability to utilize culture in the resolution of a human need.[7] I love Green's framing of the term because it puts the burden of responsibility on us. The more parochial application of cultural competence expects the disclosure of cultural information. And when they do not disclose, it lends itself to conclusions like "Well, they didn't tell me about *X, Y,* or *Z.* They should have!"

Green's definition challenges us to bear the burden of inviting culture into our interactions with the community, client, or partner. Your job is to help resolve whatever human need precipitated your interaction. Some leaders are altruistic and inherently want to help people. *Helping people is a part of the leadership role, and to be effective in that role, it's your responsibility to invite culture into this head, heart, and hands work.* For example, a physician asks the patient a simple

---

7   James Green, *Cultural Awareness in the Human Services: A Multi-Ethnic Approach* (London, UK: Pearson, 1998).

question: "What have you been doing to treat this? What did your family teach you about these types of symptoms?" From a community perspective, asking how they define the problem and what is most important to them creates avenues of dialogue that invite culture into the exchange.

When I was pregnant with Howard, I was an aerobics instructor. I had the leg warmers and the headband (it was the eighties, so everything you're imagining!) … I taught at a ladies' spa, so when recruited to teach a class for my church community, I jumped at the opportunity. I remember some of the older women in my congregation admonishing me: "You're still teaching? No, you should not be teaching!" They told me in no uncertain terms that I needed to stop. They were convinced that if I stretched and lifted my hands over my head, I ran the risk of causing the baby's umbilical cord to wrap around his neck. I was confident that their fears were unfounded, but when I started teaching the course *after* those conversations, I found myself lifting my arms a little lower than before—an example of how culture, meaning, and relationships can direct our lives and actions.

> **HELPING PEOPLE IS A PART OF THE LEADERSHIP ROLE, AND TO BE EFFECTIVE IN THAT ROLE, IT'S YOUR RESPONSIBILITY TO INVITE CULTURE INTO THIS HEAD, HEART, AND HANDS WORK.**

So many of what we call *old wives' tales* come from learned experiences. As a child, my mother once got a deep cut across her jaw—right on the bone. Her grandmother went around the house collecting cobwebs from various corner spaces and put the webs on her wound. In the telling of this story, the bleeding stopped shortly thereafter. Some natural remedies have science behind them. Just because we're unaware of the mechanism of action doesn't mean it's not valid. These may not always be scientifically based, but understand that this can carry just as much truth as the "facts" in how they shape the reactions and lives of people. These practices have relevance, or maybe not, but we can't separate anyone from their culture in terms of the specific human need that's being resolved. How do we use culture to determine a human need? How do we set a tone in which people are comfortable sharing their authentic, genuine selves, especially across difference?

We build and earn trust in various ways. Listening deeply to stories, without spoken or unspoken ridicule, can be a significant deposit in any relationship account. Those with whom we engage observe us in our encounters. For example, with the story about my mother and great-grandmother, if this story were shared with someone else and authentically received, the internal response might be "I told her that story about the cobwebs. She didn't roll her eyes or say that it made no sense!" How do we affirm for the sake of authentic communication? How can we listen to stories across difference and exclaim, "Isn't that amazing—the creativity of your great-great-grandmother!"

That is what inviting culture into problem-solving can look like. Find an authentic place to include and invite culture. How do we recognize that we have different lived experiences across race? What we seek to gain is the *richness of relationship*, and when we find the cultural overlap, that's the cherry on top. When you're "racially discordant" with someone, but still able to affirm that you've had similar experiences, you set the stage for growth and connection. Authentic communication is about earning trust—*building* trust. It's a means to healing. It also creates room at the table for everyone.

AUTHENTICITY—NOT PERFECTION!—IN CULTURAL COMPETENCE

Inter-cultural dialogue and respect for diversity are
more essential than ever in a world where peoples are
becoming more and more closely interconnected.

—KOFI ANNAN

Black children are taught as children to *see* color—out of love from their parents—often as a protective or defensive mechanism. It operates from the lived experience that *others* see race and culture and will make assumptions about our heritage. White children are raised not to see color. The motivation is likely the same: "I want you to be safe, well, and whole." And so, do or do *not* see people's race/ color and risk offending …

But seeing race can have great interpersonal and collective benefit. For years and years, my wonderful neighbor, an older white woman, has put together a Christmas village in her basement around the holidays. All the kids come and see the little houses and flickering lights. My god-grandson was visiting for the holidays one year and my neighbor extended an invitation. "Bring Montgomery over to see the Christmas village!" So we came over and saw the decorations, but my neighbor quickly pulled me to the side. "Renée, I have to tell you something. I've been putting this town up for years and years, and I didn't notice until this year that there are no Black people in my village! I'll tell you what—I'm taking care of that today!"

I don't know if my heart was more warmed by the fact that she had made the observation or that she was comfortable discussing the revelation with me! I thanked her for noticing. Isn't it amazing when you've been looking at something for years and didn't see it until you did? She told her daughter the story, and she responded, "Mom, that is so racist. I can't believe you said that to Renée! I'm sure you offended her." Then, my sweet neighbor called to tell me that she was concerned. She apologized and said she didn't mean to offend. I assured her, "There is nothing less offensive than being seen. You seeing that there were no Black people in that town was a testament to your seeing *me* and understanding that you have a Black friend who would not envision herself in that town the way it has always been."

I thanked her (1) for noticing and (2) for having the authenticity to say something. I disagreed with her daughter's reprimand. It's easier to ignore and deflect. Everyone dreads putting on those washed jeans! It's common to think, *I don't have to deal with this situation. Instead of facing it and having authentic communication and dialogue, I'll walk away.* I would submit that these moments occur all around us. My neighbor's desire for authentic relationship superseded her fear of saying the wrong thing.

Oftentimes, the experiences we have in our personal lives build the muscles for addressing such matters in our work lives, where it is the most difficult—sensitivity is elevated, if not escalated. You'll get a lot of "Well, you guys are always focused on race." Actually, I'm focused on my authentic self, and race is a part of my identity. If I had a physical disability and talked about how I'm differently abled, no one would be offended by that. No one would say, "Well, she's always talking about people who use wheelchairs, who have mobility differences." That would be a part of who I am, and no one would be offended by it.

This work is known to offend, often because of the unresolved racialized experiences in this country, which cause us not to say anything—to pretend as though no one saw it. I have white people tell me all the time that their mother, father, or family taught them that *you don't see race.* Well then, you're not seeing who *I* am. Are we taught to not see gender? No. Our relationship will be different because our gender is different—and then enriched and made more wonderful due to recognizing the difference. Likewise, our relationship will be different and enriched *because our races are different …* when you allow yourself to see it. Cultural competency, despite its detractors or naysayers, invites the recognition of difference, a skill greatly needed by equity leaders.

There are things I've experienced and learned because of my tradition and culture—practices potentially foreign to you if you are racially and culturally different from me—that could embellish and strengthen our relationship when embraced. Ironically, when so many fear being called racist, *seeing* color is an important strategy to avoid the misinterpretation of race-based exchanges. The common white American battle cry to not see or say anything about race is destructive to relationship when Black kids are taught to *see*.

> **OUR RELATIONSHIP WILL BE DIFFERENT BECAUSE OUR GENDER IS DIFFERENT—AND THEN ENRICHED AND MADE MORE WONDERFUL DUE TO RECOGNIZING THE DIFFERENCE.**

We are still striving to keep people whole on both spectrums of the racial divide. Social safety is the motivation on both sides—it simply manifests differently. Cultural competence operationalized by intentionally including culture in exchanges disarms confusion. It strips away anything that gets in the way of authentic (messy at times!) communication.

LEARNING LESSONS: AUTHENTIC COMMUNICATION

- Attend to intent and impact.
- Authentic communication comes from fully being you, and permitting others to do the same.
- Cultural competence is the ability to utilize culture in the resolution of a human need.
- *See* color, and embrace difference.

MIRROR MOMENTS: AUTHENTIC COMMUNICATION

1. When was the last time you shied away from authentic communication? What prevented you from bringing your full self to the exchange?
2. Remind yourself of an instance of authentic communication. What moved you the most in the exchange?
3. When has intent versus impact influenced an interpersonal encounter that you experienced or observed?

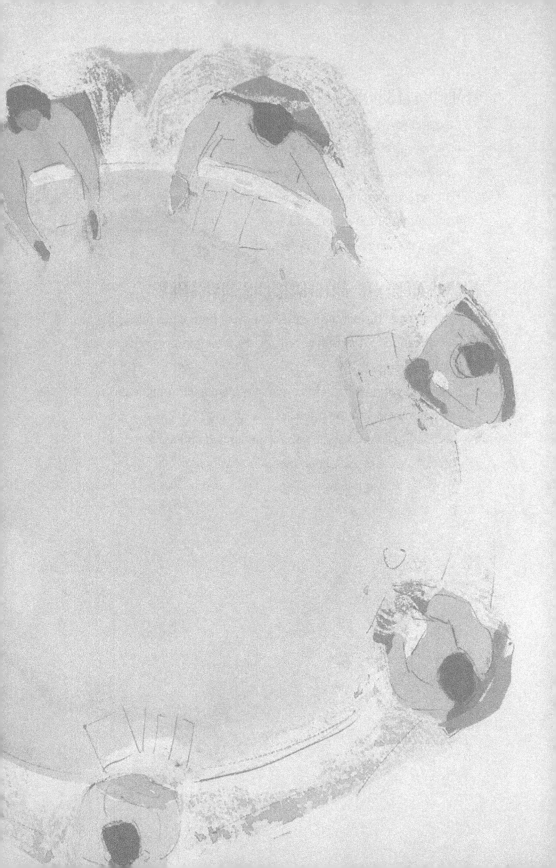

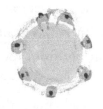

CHAPTER SIX

THE POWER OF WORDS AND WORDS OF POWER

Be careful with your words. Once they are said,
they can be only forgiven, not forgotten.

—UNKNOWN

My colleagues in community organizing taught me that power is the ability to act—in other words, the ability to effect change. Words have power; they change things. When I worked at Michigan State, I attended a funeral after the tragic and untimely death of one of my students. Somehow, I ended up being the driver of a minivan carrying four colleagues, and as we pulled into the parking lot, only two spaces remained. I said aloud, "Eeny, meeny, miny, moe …" to which someone in the back seat replied, "Catch a nigger by its toe!"

My four colleagues in the van were all white women. One person laughed out loud, and then there was muffled nervous laughter from the others in the van—but not from me. I sat frozen and replied, "That is not funny. I don't understand why you all are laughing." I looked to the woman who had ended the nursery rhyme with the disparaging—though common—phrase, as I tried to wrap my head around why she would feel comfortable saying such a thing. Thinking back, I assume her response was knee-jerk. She'd likely heard "catch a N— by the toe" so many times before.

For the record, this children's rhyme concludes with "catch a tiger by its toe."

I pulled into the parking space, and as you can imagine, there was tense discomfort throughout the minivan. Everyone hurried to get out. They walked into the church as I was still trying to gather myself. Once the ceremony was over, we returned to the van and made the journey home in complete silence. In the absence of any expression of regret or remorse, I decided it was important to notify the dean of this event and did so immediately upon our arrival on campus. The dean expressed disappointment and concern at hearing the details of this incident. The solution that she offered to this hugely disruptive event was to require that this colleague send me an emailed apology. Why was this solution equally problematic?

I often use this story as an example of the power of words with my students and ask them that question. How does this solution add to the problem rather than resolve the problem? Some students would make the point that the woman *did* apologize … But did she? Reflect again on the context of the insult that I experienced—did it take place as a private event just between me and her? No. It happened publicly in front of three other colleagues who were now left thinking, *Glad that is over* or perhaps that it was an isolated incident, limited to the offense being spoken and the awkward aftermath in the car. Perhaps they assumed, "It wasn't that big of a deal. So glad we can just move past this."

Unfortunately, we have no way of knowing what the impact was on the other people involved in this occurrence because the incident was not leveraged for healing and learning. It could have been an important teaching moment for those involved. Even if it wasn't a teaching moment for my colleagues, it can now be one for many, and that's why I use the story today. The response missed the opportunity to create authentic relationship—to advance healing. It missed the chance for cultural transformation and reiterated destructive notions without any actions to contradict them.

Had this incident occurred as a private interpersonal exchange between two people and the solution was sending a public apology to all employees, you would immediately see the ridiculousness in the response. It is similarly nonsensical to take a public event and hide the remediation in an interpersonal exchange. Not only did the event affect people in addition to the two of us who had the verbal exchange, but it also directly influenced those who observed and indirectly participated. Similarly, the reactions by those in the van as well as the dean collectively speak to the culture of the organization where such an event would so comfortably occur. Words have power, and in this case, they revealed destructive characteristics across personal attitudes, interpersonal engagements, and cultural norms. Indeed, words have power …

Retelling this story still stings. Words have influence and impact. Although this story reveals a more blatant example, there are other exchanges happening regularly with words and their context resulting in significant damage. What subtle but powerful, even if *innocent*, words are you using?

THE WORDS OF POWER—THE SILENCE OF POWER

*Let no corrupting talk come out of your mouths, but
only such as is good for building up, as fits the occasion,
that it may give grace to those who hear.*

—EPHESIANS 4:29

Words don't exist in isolation, and they don't manifest as disembodied sounds. Words must be written or spoken at the hand or mouth of a person, and oftentimes it is a person of and with power. That is you! So let's reflect on your power. I'm constantly reminding myself that regardless of our attempts to be purists, the messenger does matter. The phrase *words of power* emphasizes the words of powerful people, and the words of people of power can result in good or bad, depending on the leader's intent.

The previous story illustrates how words have power, but words are most powerful when powerful people use them *intentionally*. If you are reading this book, you have power. Leaders often think about the power of their position. But as an equity leader, *it is not about the position; it is about the positioning*. Positioning affords you the opportunity to use words of power with limited personal conse-quences, unlike others who may not hold the roles and authority of leadership. We can often speak

IT IS NOT ABOUT THE POSITION; IT IS ABOUT THE POSITIONING.

when others cannot or will not. Equity leaders should have the emotional intelligence or discernment that helps them understand that their powerful words can **make space** for others, giving voice to the voiceless. "Some things are better left unsaid" makes sense when coming from those with power and *better said* by those experiencing the conditions being discussed.

I think back to that moment in the minivan on the way to the funeral. I chose silence. Why did I do that? In many ways, my choice was an *application* of power and strength. I was outraged. I could have lashed out and skillfully dissected what had just occurred, hastily taking a scalpel to her words with no regard to whether she got cut. But I chose to use the only power I had at that moment to contain myself and wait. *Silence.* I had no positional or social power at the time. These were tenured faculty, and I was a non-tenure-track administrator. Recall also that I was the only person of color in this scenario. As an afterthought, perhaps *that* is how I ended up being the driver! Power dynamics positioned the events that transpired in that van.

As a person of power, or a leader with power, it is your responsibility to understand that the right thing can be said at the wrong time. It is not always what you say or how you say it but **when** you say it. The common phrase is "Timing is everything." There are moments when it is not about the words you choose to say. The *timing* of speaking them could have the polar-opposite impact of what you intended, even deflating everyone in the room. If you make space for strategic silence, others might also have the space to think about what happened, and perhaps your words will be empowering instead of debilitating.

I chose silence in my moment of outrage because I didn't think it was *productive* to speak out at the time. My colleagues would not have been in a position to hear … If I had lashed out, it wouldn't have left them better—it likely would have left them *bitter.* They weren't ready to grapple. The problem is often rationalized by thinking to themselves, *Oh, she's so sensitive. You can't say anything to people these days.* When discomfort is escalated at the wrong time, people go into all types of coping strategies. They're uncomfortable and fearful. They want to flee. Keeping people whole and keeping them at the table requires the right words at the right time, and words of power are determinant in such cases.

When we returned to the van, one colleague whispered, "I'm really sorry that happened." The first misplaced amend resulting from this situation … She didn't want to talk about it. She just needed to say those words. Those ladies were anxious, likely expecting the worst as they anticipated my reaction. My choice to withhold choice words (oh, I could have let them have it!) required them to think about the situation on that hour-long drive back from the funeral. Silence can be a strategic use of power, in the withholding of words. When you are strategic about the right time and place to give voice to the necessary words, you demonstrate your power in useful and constructive ways.

When striving toward this shared space of experience and maturity as leaders, we recognize that we are not all on the same timeline. Our lived experiences shape the kinds of leaders we'll be, and some of us have life-altering experiences early in our careers. Others get the trickle effect—a little thing happened here, and another happened there. These events shape us into who we are and position us to discern how to best use our words (or silence) of power.

EFFECTIVE OR AFFECTIVE LEADERSHIP— HOW WORDS ARE TOOLS FOR CONNECTION

effect:

a change that is a result or consequence of an action or other cause.

affect:

to touch the feelings of; move emotionally.

As leaders, we are socialized to focus on knowledge, information, facts, and, dare I say, evidence. But as *equity* leaders, what we provide is more than intellectual knowledge. This is *head, heart, and hands work!* What do your heart and emotions tell you is the right thing to do and the right time to do it? What is most needful, more so than what is necessary? Needful speaks to the desire for, or the pursuit of, something that is missing. Needful is an urgent want for something requisite. More than impacting the mind by adding more knowledge or facts, how do we impress the mind or *push* our minds to shape an opinion about facts and information?

It is an obvious truth that equity is necessary (essential, indispensable, and requisite), and as equity leaders, our goal is to see equity become a necessary component of our work and lives, but as of now, that state is wanting. You cannot be effective as an equity leader without attending to the *affective*—without being concerned with the emotions and feelings that underpin your action or inaction for equity. Your feelings and emotions shape the power you hold, and the power you hold shapes the words that create policy, change, and healing. Your lived experiences summon and shape your affective stance. Think for a moment about the semantic dance between these words and phrases: effect or affect; the power of words and the words of power. Again, if you are not an *affective* leader, you will not be an effective leader because you are not using all the frames and mental models available to you. Affective leaders see people and meet them at the point of their needs because of their awareness of feelings and opinions.

In our equity workshops at MPHI titled Advancing Justice Together (ADJUST), we have an exercise called "What's in a name?" It reminds me of the rumination in this speech from Shakespeare's Romeo and Juliet:

O! be some other name:
What's in a name? that which we call a rose
By any other name would smell as sweet.

Juliet wishes for Romeo to *not* be a Montague because of an endless family feud. I say, "Juliet, just call him by his name!" His name still represents the essence of who he is; calling him something else does not change who he is. The flower called a rose is still the same flower even if called a hose! But if you are mindful of what's in a name and the frames you shape by the words you choose, then you center *people*, as opposed to centering problems. We must be more conscious of this than ever before. It is the hallmark of an *affective* equity leader.

> **IF YOU ARE MINDFUL OF WHAT'S IN A NAME AND THE FRAMES YOU SHAPE BY THE WORDS YOU CHOOSE, THEN YOU CENTER PEOPLE, AS OPPOSED TO CENTERING PROBLEMS.**

We sometimes get in our way when seeking to center people and honor the heart of equity work. That was the case for my journey as a cisgender heterosexual woman to understand the shift to *identify* and expand the use of pronouns. My discomfort drove me to find any and every reason why we shouldn't use our pronouns, as is now an increasingly common practice in many settings. I went from "Doesn't asking people to introduce themselves with their pronouns 'out' those who may not use binary pronouns? Or does it force them to fake their pronouns if the space is not safe?" Although my words suggested that I was centering the community most impacted, leaning into the affective aspects "outed" me and my own discomfort. That recognition and self-awareness is always the first step in growth.

Words of power (from me!) converted my discomfort … But if my use of my pronouns as a person with power indicates to others my desire to center the unique needs of others, especially others who are different from me, then it was on me to increase my comfort with discomfort. And ultimately, discomfort be gone! That took a great deal of self-reflection (my own Mirror Moment). If you want to be in authentic relationship with others, to inspire them to be their best, then you must sincerely consider who they are. Equity leaders carry themselves in a way that demonstrates trustworthiness through what they do and say. No matter where you're positioned, involving the people most impacted by the decisions you make or the problems you must solve is most effective. Acknowledge the *affective* feelings and emotions that may be barriers to that goal.

As a leader and person with power, you will observe the impact of power on relationships, including efforts by staff to distance themselves from power. An implicit way this often manifests is the tendency for people to reify organizational and departmental partners (this habit is a personal pet peeve of mine!). I am sure you've heard it before: "The department won't let us do that" or "The division said we have to turn the report in today." And I consequently ask, "Who? *Who* said that?" And when the response is "the department," I use all my appreciation for relationship to control frustration or leaning into sarcasm. I have trouble hearing about what the "division" has to say because the last time I checked, the "division" doesn't have a brain or mouth! I can't pick up the phone and have a nice conversation with the "division." I'd be talking at a building. I can have a conversation with *someone who works* in the division. Oftentimes, this kind of language is just about getting out of something (a form of words/ silence of power)—"The department said we can't" or "The university said they won't, so let's move on."

While acknowledging the affective, equity leadership under-stands the power of words to center *people* and the *words of power* that center people. The depth of the problem is revealed in subtle ways. Consider the common response to those from cultures that are different from your own whose names are "hard to pronounce." Hard to pronounce for whom? I'm certain it is not difficult for them to say their own name, or hard for their parents, relatives, and people who love them to say their name. All too often we center ourselves in these moments—"I don't want to say their name wrong, so let's just shorten it." *Saying* someone's name is powerful—*hearing* your name is powerful. Rather than hoping to be let off the hook with a nickname, how do we require ourselves to apply our power in ways that honor the names of the people with whom we are in relationship? Lest you get distracted, this example, in this context, is about the use of power. Intentionality about words and power can solidify or weaken relationship. An affective equity leader knows what's in a name.

LISTENING—THE CATALYST FOR YOUR WORDS

generalization:

a general statement or concept obtained by inference from specific cases.

stereotype:

a widely held but fixed and oversimplified image or idea of a particular type of person or thing.

Once upon a time, someone thought it wise to say, "There's no such thing as a stupid question." I beg to differ! Nothing could be further from the truth. You've heard them—the questions that clearly reveal that the person has not been listening at all to the discussion that preceded their question. The fuel for the power of words and words of power is listening. Let's look deeper …

Listening often determines whether we land at a generalization or a stereotype. Generalizations are the start of the story, and stereotypes are the conclusion. Consider this scenario. For the purposes of this scenario, you are a nutritionist and have "heard" that Black families from the south eat a lot of fried food. You meet Mrs. Johnson, who happens to be an African American woman from the south, and you could *conclude* that she must eat a lot of fried food. You have placed yourself at the end of Mrs. Johnson's story without listening or learning. What you do with the information determines whether it reinforces a stereotype ("southern Blacks eat a lot of fried food") or whether it informs the initiation of the relationship ("I wonder if Mrs. Johnson eats a diet of mostly fried food")—a generalization that must be vetted to see if it is true in this case.

> **LISTENING OFTEN DETERMINES WHETHER WE LAND AT A GENERALIZATION OR A STEREOTYPE. GENERALIZATIONS ARE THE START OF THE STORY, AND STEREOTYPES ARE THE CONCLUSION.**

Perhaps Mrs. Johnson is obese, so you think, *She eats a lot of fried food because I know she's from the south.* That is the conclusion to the story, and again, a stereotype. But if you're talking with Mrs. Johnson and make no assumptions based upon the information you have, as a nutritionist you might say, "Talk to me about your diet," and she replies, "Well, we bake or grill our meats, and I'm trying to eat less meat …" Even though she's from the south, her response contradicts the information you have, serving more as a generalization that started your encounter.

Certainly, there are patterns across cultures and among people. For sociologists, the meat and potatoes—pardon the pun—of what we study are patterns, collective behaviors, and social norms. We know that cultures and group norms often express themselves in shared behaviors, but just because there is a collective pattern, it doesn't mean it is true for a particular individual. There's that ecological fallacy concept again! Just because it is true for the collective doesn't mean that it is true for the individual. And just because it's true for the individual doesn't mean you will see that across the collective.

We all make generalizations, but stereotypes are more likely to be destructive, even stereotypes that are "favorable." Consider the concept of the "ideal minority," often applied to Asian Americans. It sounds like this: "Oh, you're Asian. You must be great at math." It seems like a compliment, but it is instead a stereotype (assumed as true without any evidence). Many people of Asian descent do not excel at math. Even uttering those words causes extra social pressure on individuals to perform or to "represent their race." I admire Spanish-speaking cultures and have studied Spanish throughout high school and college, but I cannot presume that everyone I meet with a Latinx name speaks Spanish without vetting, hearing, and learning directly from the person.

During my time serving in the College of Nursing, there seemed to be an era of textbooks that tried to be culturally progressive. You can easily spot them because there is the telltale African American chapter, Asian American chapter, Hispanic American chapter, etc.… I have even seen some books that lean into this model and also include white ethnic groups, like a Polish American chapter or Italian American chapter.

Having reviewed several such texts, I will confess that I have never read a Black chapter that represented my lived experiences. Sometimes, as I'm reading, I have to ask myself, "Who did they interview for their information?" I recall reviewing a chapter on African Americans that described Blacks as very religious, including the common practice of voodoo. If someone came up to me and said, "Oh, you're Black. You must practice voodoo. Talk to me about it," imagine what that statement would do to our relationship. Cultural knowledge is important, but using information and knowledge to stereotype or overgeneralize offers another example of the power of words to harm.

Generalizations can be a starting point for listening. Then if the people you are talking to offer lived expriences that uphold the information you have read, you have a context from which to build relationship. Listening is a vital skill to build authentic relationship across cultures. Silence becomes the catalyst for choosing your words. In many ways, our silence and listening hold equal importance across our words of power. In many power-based relationships, our listening is a stance of strength, even when we are socialized to enter the space as experts with all the knowledge and facts. "You're the leader, so come in prepared to talk." Resist that urge, and come in prepared to listen so that you can channel your power in meaningful and equitable ways.

LEARNING LESSONS: THE POWER OF WORDS AND WORDS OF POWER

- Words have the power to harm or heal.
- In recognizing words of power, we recognize that we have power.
- Aim to be an affective leader.
- Generalizations are the beginning of the story, and stereotypes are the conclusion.
- Listening is the catalyst for your words.

MIRROR MOMENTS: THE POWER OF WORDS AND WORDS OF POWER

1. Recall a time when someone said something to you that hit you "like a ton of bricks." You deeply felt the power of words.
2. Now, recall when you used the words of power! What did that feel like? Was the outcome good or bad?
3. Name a stereotype you still hold onto. If you don't have one, name a stereotype that someone else holds on to. How can you shift your thinking, or that of others, about this stereotype? Remind yourself of an instance of authentic communication. What moved you the most in the exchange?
4. When has intent versus impact influenced an interpersonal encounter that you experienced or observed?

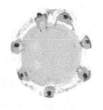

CHAPTER SEVEN

BUILDING RELATIONSHIP FOR EQUITY

Relationships are primary; all else is derivative.

—RON DAVID, MD

Think about a time when you were aware of your difference. In other words, think about a time when you were in a space or place and knew you were not the same as others. It may have been a situation as simple as going to an after-work party that you thought was business casual or "come as you are." Upon arriving, you realized that it turned out to be a fancy cocktail party. Looking around at the semiformal attire, you see it is very clear that you are different.

While I typically do this exercise in a group, I invite you to reflect on what the incident was and why you were different in that setting. If you cannot think of a time when you felt different, challenge yourself to create a future moment. There are people in our society who wake up every day, open their doors, and walk out into difference.

Now, more important than the occasion, I invite you to think about how that incident made you feel. In my thirty-year career, I have probably asked this question thousands of times in workshops and training, and I can count on one hand when the responses were things like "Oh, I felt special, unique, valued, and important," etc. You catch my drift. People consistently share feelings like "I felt awkward, out of place, uncomfortable, angry, and confused. I felt like I stood out." Perhaps you see your feelings among these. The sentiments are consistently on the negative side of Gloria Wilcox's feelings wheel. This demonstrates another pattern in how we live our lives in the United States. There is something about the experience of being different that is uncomfortable and difficult.

We say we value *diversity*, but we shun *difference*. In many ways we truly do not want to be different—we deeply wish to avoid difference and pretend like we are all the same! Initially, this was frustrating for me. If we say we value diversity and differences, it would seem that we would somehow feel excited when faced with our own difference or that of others—but that doesn't typically appear to be the case. Perhaps somewhere in our personal reactions to difference, there is the hint of a deep desire to connect, even when we are not the same—to embrace our similarities and commonalities. What do we share with those who are different? *What are the ties that bind us?*

Difference has often been a barrier to building relationship, rather than an enhancement for new relationships. Instead of seeing difference through a polarized lens (either we are different or we are the same), seek out similarities or differences that you can relate to or learn from. If you're talking with someone from a different culture or community than yours and ask, "What is your favorite holiday tradition?" and the response is something familiar or similar to yours—even though you are both "different"—you have found an on-ramp to relationship! You connect … *We're all looking for what we can connect on, but we can seek out commonality while also embracing difference.* Imagine a conversation that sounds like this: "That experience sounds so great. We have the same tradition, but we do it a little differently in our family."

How do we develop a culture that is not intimidated or threatened by difference but instead truly embraces it? How do we sacrifice our deep investment in sameness? As teachers, physicians, public health professionals, friends, or parents, we should not treat the people we serve the same. *What?* That sounds like sacrilege! Case in point: "I treat all my patients the same; I treat all my students the same; I treat all my clients the same," etc.—these are not relationship goals! Too often in this work we hear the phrase "I'm not racist. I treat all people the same." Therein lies the problem! We are not all the same, so why would we set treating everyone the same as the gold standard? That is an equality mindset that heals no one and does nothing to help us build relationships for equity.

> **WE'RE ALL LOOKING FOR WHAT WE CAN CONNECT ON, BUT WE CAN SEEK OUT COMMONALITY WHILE ALSO EMBRACING DIFFERENCE.**

We must lean into the truth that it is okay to be, treat, or see people differently. The offhanded comment (which I have heard on more than one occasion) that "when I see you, Renée, I don't see a Black person" is as insulting as the backhanded compliment (which I have also heard on more than one occasion) that "you are really pretty, for a Black girl." Not seeing someone as a Black person or distorting your seeing of a Black person is nothing to brag about. To get comfortable as a leader who drives equity in your field, you've got to look for and seek out difference. (1) Recognize it, (2) celebrate it, and (3) figure out what you need to do differently as a result of it.

There is very little that we accomplish outside of relationship. It is primary, and all else derives from it. *Difference as uniqueness is a strength ...* and a relationship asset. Make peace with difference. That's where equity begins to blossom.

THE "MAGIC NUMBER" IN DIVERSITY—THE ANTITHESIS TO BUILDING RELATIONSHIP

It's hard to keep an open mind if you don't have an open heart. You don't have to agree with what people think to learn from how they think. You don't have to share their identity to be curious about what shaped it. Treating people with civility is a prerequisite for discovery.

—ADAM GRANT

All too often, the diversity goal replicates the population demographics. For example, if the "minority" population of a city is 22 percent, a company may seek to employ 22 percent "minority" staff. That frame invites a problematic check-the-box attitude. "Okay, well, good! We've met our goal for minority staff." Not quite ... *What are the background, context, values, and simply the humanity of those employed?* Matching percentages or hitting some magical number is transactional. The goal of equity leaders is to arrive at a space that is less transactional and more relational.

WHAT ARE THE BACKGROUND, CONTEXT, VALUES, AND SIMPLY THE HUMANITY OF THOSE EMPLOYED?

Who are the people that make up the 22 percent, or the 78 percent for that matter? Who are we talking about?

I was involved in a hiring experience that demonstrates that we must think deeper than math alone. In this case, we sought out a leader who was skilled in dealing with disparities, equity, and justice. The hiring panel identified two finalists for the position—one was a white woman, and one was a Latinx man. The search committee couldn't decide who to hire. I was asked to weigh in on their dilemma. "Well, what do you think?" They wanted me to tell them what to do, to make the final decision on whom to hire. Instead, I suggested that they do one more round of interviews exclusively focused on issues of equity and justice and the candidates' experiences in that space. Then I would be happy to join the final interview.

The interview panel comprised one person of color and two white people—my inclusion balance would certainly comprise two people of color. At the end of the interview, it was so clear who the best candidate was, not because they were male or female, not because they were white or Latinx, but because one had much more knowledge and experience in the desired area. In this case, the experience elevated the Latinx applicant. The interview team's initial hesitance to select the candidate ironically sprung from a fear that people would think they had hired a Latinx male for the sake of appearances, when in fact, he was more qualified. The other expressed hesitance was concern about the "accent" that the applicant had and whether the community would be able to relate to him. Yes, this is a true story ...

The experience disturbed me, but in this case, stepping back and doing an after-action review of the process and outcome helped broaden the perspective of those on the panel. Important questions! What are we measuring when we take into account race? In this society, it may be an indicator of a shared social experience (likely experiences of oppression or resilience), but these again can be an initial positioning of the relationship that is only affirmed or debunked when deepening our interactions. In this case, the white applicant could have grown up in Black-adjacent spaces, perhaps a major metropolitan city or living her formative years in deep relationship with a diverse and inclusive community. The Latinx male could have just as easily grown up in a wealthy suburban area with little exposure to diverse populations who shared his cultural heritage. There is no space for typecasting in this work.

Equity leaders resist the urge to allow assumptions to rule the day and instead allow deep relationship to set the way forward— deep relationship that identifies great strengths, quality, expertise, and background. Difference does not have to be a roadblock. Instead, it can open the journey, pathway, and entrance ramp for authentic relationships. If you are just looking at numbers, you're missing the true potential that lies across difference.

HOW DO YOU INVITE DIFFERENCE AND INTENTIONALITY TO DIVERSITY?

> *Eating is so intimate. It's very sensual. When you invite*
> *someone to sit at your table and you want to cook for*
> *them, you're inviting a person into your life.*
>
> —MAYA ANGELOU

Maya Angelou makes a very literal point about bringing people to the table! I invite you to do the same; make a new friend. Adults aren't always encouraged to make friends. But go make a friend with someone who is different from you—who's lived differently, looks differently, and prefers different things—so that this big boulder of difference that blocks authentic relationships can be moved out of the way. I am not recommending that we bulldoze and bust up the boulders. Just set it aside as a monument to remember all that we have overcome in building authentic relationship, all the discomfort that we traversed in order to become more comfortable … Let's not forget when difference was not our friend.

You know that as a child in a military family, I was always excited when it was time for us to move to the next base assignment. Every two or three years, I got to be the new kid and sit at new tables to make friends! Discussing this with my older brother, I learned that his experience was quite different. As he described, it would take him two years to make one friend before it was time to move again. How we respond to difference in ourselves and others is unique and varied. *Authentic relationship through the equity lens helps us see that what we think is beautiful and powerful may be painful and horrid for someone else. But holding a container that allows safe and brave discussions eliminates assumptions about those around us.* I will never again assume that people who relocate, for whatever reason—business, career, or military endeavors—are having a wonderful experience just because I did. It is a difficult transition for some. I would not have had that revelation had I not leaned into authentic relationship with my brother and asked. Asking invites difference.

AUTHENTIC RELATIONSHIP THROUGH THE EQUITY LENS HELPS US SEE THAT WHAT WE THINK IS BEAUTIFUL AND POWERFUL MAY BE PAINFUL AND HORRID FOR SOMEONE ELSE. BUT HOLDING A CONTAINER THAT ALLOWS SAFE AND BRAVE DISCUSSIONS ELIMINATES ASSUMPTIONS ABOUT THOSE AROUND US.

There is an Old Testament story about the children of Israel collecting and stacking stones as a memorial—a monument placed at key stages of their journey together. I experienced a contemporary version of this practice when touring the caves of Kentucky during a family vacation with my sons. We entered Mammoth Cave and journeyed deeper and deeper into the earth. Far underground (as we leaned into the claustrophobic discomfort), what did we find? Stones stacked into a cairn, just like the children of Israel had done in the Old Testament. *Exploration*: equity is indeed a journey as well as a destination. If we remember to *remember*, we are less likely to get discouraged and lose sight of our destination or the tests and successes we experience on the way.

In addition to the visual beauty of the assembled cairns, the story behind their placement in the Kentucky caves held one additional reminder. Our tour guide shared that the stacks of rocks were the product of the creativity of enslaved people who served as tour guides in the 1800s (Stephen Bishop became a tour guide in 1838, later gaining his freedom in 1856). Our tour guide continued to share that the enslaved people told the tourists that they could add to the cairn for a small fee. After collecting their coins, the Black tour guides helped guests find a stone and add it to the monument. I'd say they designed a pretty innovative revenue-generating strategy for themselves!

However, who sets the table and tells the story matters. After our tour, I confronted difference in an unexpected way when I came across a very different narrative of this story as I flipped through a book in the gift shop. While I was excited to come across a picture of the cairn surrounded—a Black tour guide and several white tourists—I was taken aback to read the alternative narrative that instead attributed the creativity to the *tourists* as they established a tradition of adding to the growing monument of stone.

Inviting, or perhaps *discovering*, difference can help reveal truths or uncover untruths. In this case, the difference in stories had a lasting impact and serves as a reminder—or perhaps a warning. What are the monuments are we building? What are the stories they tell or the relationships they represent? What are the reminders that we should keep on this journey? What stories of difference are shaping our relationships?

SETTING A CULTURE—LEANING INTO DIFFERENCE

Therefore, having put away falsehood, let each one of you speak the truth with his neighbor, for we are members one of another.

—EPHESIANS 4:25

Culture is birthed out of relationship from which common practices and norms are established, much like the practice of setting a table for guests. You have a unique role in this as an equity leader—you set the culture and tone. Active equity culture resists the tendency to bow to the traditional "We always do it this way, and we never do it that way" worldview.

But even those old tropes turn into opportunities for building authenticity. Equity leaders challenge the status quo. *Sure, we don't do it that way, but why not? Let's see what happens if we approach it in a new way.* I like to push against the saying "If it ain't broke, don't fix it" with "If it ain't broke, fix it!" Numerous things still work, like a corded landline or an old Rolodex address file, but if it can be done more efficiently and effectively, then let's fix it! I watch my team and try to not only set an example for them but also *glean* examples from them. What do I see in their interactions and engagements that I want to replicate? The burden is not always on me—or you—to be the one who knows exactly how to respond and speak. There are brilliant people all around me, so what am I learning by engaging them in the questions and problems at hand?

This practice has been especially important as I recruited and built an effective senior leadership team. I noticed early on as a senior leader that it is very easy to recruit women who mirror my demographic and credentials. I sometimes jokingly describe myself as a brilliant-Black-woman magnet! I am certain that I could easily have built an executive team exclusively comprising doctorally prepared Black women because I am in deep relationship with those whom I have a lot in common with. I have wondered if that is the dynamic among leaders who are white men who surround themselves by a team that looks exactly like them. As an equity leader, setting an example for all leaders in my organization, leaning into difference is not optional; it is obligatory for the culture and tone I have set. And it is necessary to build relationships that will advance equity. It is not the path of least resistance or the status quo, go-with-the-flow route. Intentionality requires me to look inward and challenge my own assumptions while looking externally to create a system that includes the conditions necessary for equity to flourish.

> THERE ARE DAYS WHEN I FEEL I AM TRANSPARENT TO A FAULT, BUT THERE ARE OTHER DAYS WHEN I IMAGINE THAT TRANSPARENCY CANNOT BE A FAULT.

Building relationships for equity is an intentional effort, and the transparency of the leader is a vital asset. *There are days when I feel I am transparent to a fault, but there are other days when I imagine that transparency cannot be a fault.* If I'm true to myself, then others receive a true version of me. I am not trying to pretend. It should be natural to say, "I'm not in a space to comment just yet. I'm not certain. I need to consider this." Or my all-time favorite: simply saying, "I don't know." These responses are far more authentic and transparent than whatever results from the self-talk of "I have to come up with something to say because they're expecting me to say something. I can't let them know that I don't know." The people in the room are likely in a similar headspace as you. So inviting difference, in the form of different opinions and perspectives, helps you learn from those at the table and certainly those in the room.

I am sure you are aware of the facial expression of deep thinking—you know, furrowed brow and pensive eyes. Experience will help you pick up on when some people in the room are thinking loudly! You can practically hear their words rolling around in their brains as you observe their nonverbals. They're ready to make that "drop the mic" comment in the meeting, but will they be courageous enough to do it?! That is the precise time to learn from those who are different—to listen deeply and to make space for difference. Let's all be mindful of the boulders that can either obstruct progress or memorialize progress. Give yourself permission to imagine the monuments we will build as we progress along the journey together.

LEARNING LESSONS: BUILDING RELATIONSHIPS FOR EQUITY

- *Leaning in* is the antidote to fearing difference.
- Diversity is more than a number.
- *Invite* difference by establishing relationships with those who are different.
- You set the culture and tone for your team—observe, affirm, and listen to those around you.

MIRROR MOMENTS: BUILDING RELATIONSHIPS FOR EQUITY

1. Think of a time when you were aware of your difference. How did it make you feel?
2. Also think about a time when you observed someone else's experience of difference. How did it make you feel?
3. Put yourself out there in a situation where you are different! Go to an LGTBQ+ bar if you are straight, or if you're a white Catholic, go to a Black Baptist church. Go somewhere to intentionally be the one who is different ...

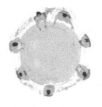

CHAPTER EIGHT

THE COURAGEOUS CHANGE

The cost of liberty is less than the price of repression.

—W. E. B. DU BOIS

L eading through equity principles can be fraught with both wariness and weariness. There are leaders who feel like they have to say the words *racial equity*, *health equity*, *antiracism*, etc., although they do so cautiously and warily on guard for the worst. I have observed people hiding behind words; they say the words, hoping nothing further will come of it—that they will get credit for saying the words without actually doing the work. In their heart of hearts, they want to check the box and move on to the next thing. When faced with this behavior, I have to fight off cynicism because I realize that many leaders don't truly understand what they're saying when they use these terms. They can say the words, but they are in no way fluent in the language of racial healing and in many ways are simply hiding behind the words.

It is easy to let "equity" work deteriorate into a pile of *words, words, words*, as Shakespeare said. The negligence of action in so many of the spaces where I serve leaves me weary, even wanting to resign or throw in the towel, but I am reminded that my voice is needed. So, deep breath and move forward! These moments of equity fatigue and fear should be indicators for action. They should force us to ask ourselves, "Right now, will I be courageous? Will I speak up?" Rather than leaning into weariness, I have endeavored to unpack the wariness that I am experiencing as well as the wariness that I am observing in others. What is causing the air of cautiousness? Why am I on guard, and how can I overcome this hesitance?

Often, you just don't have the emotional strength to speak courageously, but when a door of utterance has been opened or when a moment of silence is beckoning you to fill it, how can we as equity leaders refuse? What am I wary of at that moment? Engaging in moments of racialized tension can cause us to put up our defenses. Effortful coping in these situations can breed weariness and fatigue, which then threaten to shut down dialogue. As we strive to keep people whole and keep them at the table, are we willing to convert our wariness into a strategy to understand the wariness of others, then to prohibit it from stopping our progress?

That strategy requires both courage and change because unpacking our hesitance and fear is not a common practice. I hold a deep appreciation for the quote "The only thing necessary for evil to triumph in the world is for good people to do nothing," loosely attributed to Edmund Burke. Despite our fear and hesitance, we cannot be weary of well-doing. Courageous change does require conviction and self-negotiation. Convince yourself to resist the temptation to cease. If you are an equity leader (aspiring or existing), you simply must make the effort, even in the face of perceived backlash.

FROM BANDWAGON TO SOAPBOX

bandwagon:

used in reference to an activity, cause, etc. that is currently fashionable or popular and attracting increasing support; to change your opinion to one that has become very popular so that you can share in the success.

I like to describe it as "the Cool Kids Phenomenon." All the cool kids seem to be saying *health equity*, so others assume they had better join them. *Fashionable* and *popular* are not authentic or sincere. As I penned this chapter, I considered another wearying situation that was fresh in my mind. I facilitated a health agency through its antioppression journey. They were engaged in a hiring process at the time. I reviewed their staff demographics and commented on the lack of diversity—I was not advocating for a quota mindset (remember, it is not a numbers game) but inquired how they were mindful of *presence and representation* in their process.

The person they ended up hiring was white, and they proceeded to assure me that she was highly qualified. I informed them that my guidance was in no way an indictment of the caliber of the new staff member and asked them to reflect on why they came to that erroneous interpretation of my question. Certainly, she must be qualified if she was hired. The committee's defense of their choice, in my mind, was akin to a parent proclaiming, "I feed my kids every day." Of course you do! My agitation was intended to push them to reflect on the fact that their qualified applicant pool included no people of color. My grievance stemmed from the process and foundation—you can't have a diverse qualified workforce without an applicant pool that mirrors those characteristics. *Looking deeper, I wondered why exactly they didn't have a diverse qualified applicant pool.* I saw the exchange shift from the cool kids on the bandwagon to minimizing my comments to that of a soapbox. Yes, perhaps I was speaking of something that I felt strongly about, but I also saw them using that same passion to minimize and discount the points I was making.

I could hear their loud thinking and unspoken words—*here comes Renée on her soapbox again.* Yet still, equity leadership demands that we speak in these moments when courageous change is necessary. We want to be on an organizational equity journey, but we don't want to diversify our workforce? It may be true that you want to be on an equity journey, but the fact is you really don't want to do the work to diversify your workforce (again, getting equity credit without doing the work). I challenge you in your equity leadership role to keep yourself accountable for dissecting the contradictions to equity in any situation while illuminating the *reasons* why change is vital. Equity leaders can pursue courageous change despite the weariness and wariness that stifle action.

THE WARRIOR CHILD—BATTLING FOR EQUITY

Lately I've been winning battles left and right
But even winners can get wounded in the fight
People say that I'm amazing
Strong beyond my years
But they don't see inside of me
I'm hiding all the tears
They don't know that I go running home when I fall down
They don't know who picks me up when no one is around
I drop my sword and cry for just a while

'Cause deep inside this armor
The warrior is a child.

—TWILA PARIS, "THE WARRIOR IS A CHILD"

It is not uncommon for those who do not experience racism to see it as a problem of Black people (or BIPOC). Racism is not a *people of color* problem. It is a *people* problem, whether Black, Indigenous, Asian, Latinx, or white. Similarly, leading through equity principles is for all leaders—not just a strategy for BIPOC leaders. Courageous change also isn't solely intended for people of color, but you will see this misunderstanding everywhere. That is why courageous dialogue is more important than ever. In the face of "You're calling me a racist" (I've told you about this accusation, and you've likely heard this accusation … It won't stop soon enough), don't allow that all-to-common comment to end the conversation and prevent equity dialogue from advancing. There is a great benefit to courageously leaning into these moments for the sake of change—for the sake of opening minds and hearts.

The practice of keeping people whole and keeping them at the table requires a level of selflessness when confronted with racialized moments or incidents. I have found that the simplest of comments can be overinterpreted and overpersonalized in shallow ways. The truth is, the comment "Don't take this personally" can't be further from the truth. We absolutely do need leaders to take growth opportunities personally. Intent versus impact only works if we take the moment personally and determine its applicability to ourselves.

I recall on more than one occasion facilitating dialogue about racism when someone made the statement "I feel like you are saying I'm a racist" or "But I'm not a racist." While the natural inclination may be defensiveness and a desire to shut down the dialogue, the goal is to advance change by keeping the dialogue open. Instead of strongly correcting them with "I did not call you a racist," my goal is to keep dialogue open with a more thoughtful response when it seems that someone is trying to get up from the table:

- "Let's unpack your comment."
- "Can you say a little more?"
- "Let's discuss that point further."

And of course, a sincere apology goes a long way to keep people at the table: "I'm so sorry you felt that I called you a racist" or "I take responsibility for the impact of my actions or words even when they were not my intent." As we keep the dialogue open, people figure out pretty soon that it's not the words they are hearing—it's the self-talk in their heads. Many people are immediately operating on all cylinders once they hear the terms *equity, racism, oppression, BIPOC, LGBTQ+,* etc.

All too often, we see words or terms commonly used in the public equity narrative weaponized and applied in completely counterintuitive ways. The phrase *social justice warrior* has been co-opted and weaponized in some settings to be a disparaging label. Yet, training and preparing warriors for social justice and equity are exactly why we lead in this space. Ironically, *warrior* is defined as a person who has great vigor or courage. Courage is the fuel for social justice

TIMING YOUR WORDS IS STRATEGIC, BUT WITHHOLDING YOUR WORDS IS COWARDICE.

warriors, to build strength (muscles) and instinct (heart) for this work. After a while, you know you can and *must* lean into controversy. Nonetheless, with your commitment to being a change agent and equity leader, you realize that withdrawal is not an option. But you can pause, you can pace yourself … *Timing your words is strategic, but withholding your words is cowardice.*

Our job is to be vulnerable and transparent knowing that we are bolstered by equity values. For many reasons, people avoid taking risks in tense moments. They have another life—a separate life. We are taught to stay in a compartmentalized world where there is a work self and a personal self. It's easy to step back and avoid situations when your work self is grappling with difficult moments. Why? Because you can run home to be your *personal* self, where you're loved, valued, and affirmed—and can vent.

As a change agent, we return to the *proper* life balance, no longer running away from the equity challenges we may face in the workplace. When you stop running, you set an example for others to also stop running. I would submit that we've been running from our work selves way too long in this society. We've allowed the myth of the *professional* and *personal* to disrupt progress in many spaces, but particularly the space of racialized relationships, which then undergirds racialized institutions and, ultimately, buttresses a racialized culture. Having the courage to speak the truth in your leadership role—in your work environment—is direct and courageous action against the social forces that suggest that we do otherwise. With this freedom to be our whole selves in an equity-driven space, we see transformation. *The social justice warrior becomes the equity victor.*

AND AS ALWAYS, TO STEP AWAY AND TAKE A BREATH IS HUMAN (AND HEALTHY), BUT TO RETURN WITH THE RIGHT WORDS AT THE RIGHT TIME IS COURAGEOUS.

Courageous change, leaning in, and bringing your full self—these actions stem from habit, from building that muscle until you don't notice the muscle anymore. The more you do it, the more you do it! I want to agitate conviction in you because, like any other human in this work, many want to leave the table. Equity leaders instigate difficult conversations and foment "good trouble," a remarkable phrase used by John Lewis. *And as always, to step away and take a breath is human (and healthy), but to return with the right words at the right time is courageous.*

Many leaders are resigned and believe that we have made sufficient progress and things are good enough. "It's not as bad as it used to be. The boxes are checked so that no one needs to lean in. Everyone can go home." You know my motto; say it with me: Good enough is not good enough! Equity work is fluid and ongoing, beckoning everyone to join. Courageous equity work can become a part of our culture—our society—once it is modeled, demonstrated, and, ultimately, normalized.

In our ADJUST (Advancing Justice Together) workshop at MPHI, we champion the fact that *dialogue is doing; facilitated dialogue is a methodology for action*. It is a methodology for change. In staff meetings, I have used the prompt, "Who was courageous this week and how?" When posing this question, I'm looking for stories of courage that might be as simple as telling your mother you're not coming home for Thanksgiving!

After someone shares their brave moment, we can then unpack their experience by asking, "Well, how did you get the nerve?" They might answer that instead of seeing their mother for the holidays, another valuable experience called to them. They had to make a choice … And maybe their mother was upset, but just for a moment. The relationship might have grown even stronger because of the expression of honesty! It was not as hard or as bad as they anticipated.

This simple exercise highlights what courage *feels* like and reminds them that courage is not space dependent … Eventually, those in the meeting begin to recognize that gut sensation, and it opens a door to courageous change in other spaces. No, it's not easy. There will be days when you feel more like the child than the warrior in the lyrics to Twila Paris's song, but as she said, "the warrior is a child." We are both the professional social warrior and the personal innocent child, combining immaculately to build the muscle for courage and change.

THE BEAUTY OF TAKING RISKS—COURAGE IN ACTION

Whatever actions you take, keep in mind that over the course of life, you will fail far more from timidity, procrastination, and carefulness than you will from just stepping up to the plate and, as we say in Australia, giving it a bloody go!

—MARGIE WARRELL

I vividly recall reaching a point where my impatience with cowardly leaders boiled over. I sat in various meetings over an extended season and listened as leaders chose silence rather than speaking up when faced with matters of inequity. In other scenarios, leaders soft-pedaled or deflected the discussion. Observing this recurring pattern made me wonder what was causing these otherwise effective leaders to cower in the face of potential opposition or resistance. Frequently, these discussions that prompted "non-responses" addressed matters that would necessitate change—something needed to happen, a shift or variation to disrupt the status quo. *Overcoming the resistance of others requires that you overcome the hesitance of yourself.*

> OVERCOMING THE RESISTANCE OF OTHERS REQUIRES THAT YOU OVERCOME THE HESITANCE OF YOURSELF.

Processing such hesitance is an equity skill, a skill that acknowledges the affective impact of change. I'll share an applied example. Recently, the pastor of my church announced his resignation, and I cochaired the "transition team." There had been plenty of chatter prior to the meeting based on the information (or misinformation) that committee members had heard. We opened our meeting by asking everyone to think about a time when they were involved in a significant change.

Many told stories about a new job, a move, a change in companionship, and more examples, but all could remember an incident where change had affected them directly. In processing the responses to this question, we did not ask for specifics about the context of their stories; rather, I asked them to describe their *feelings* associated with this moment of change. How did it feel to be in the midst of the change? Most shared that they were worried, nervous, fearful, frustrated, or unsure. Only one said that they were peaceful.

It is illuminating that the very idea of change prompts these reactions; even when it is a *good* change ("I'm so sick of this job and want a new one!"), it often makes people nervous, anxious, and worried. It is a tough truth, but change often precipitates tough emotions. Avoiding tough emotions is also a common reaction, and perhaps that is what contributes to behaviors that can be categorized as cowardly in the context of meeting the needs of equity change. But what does it feel like *on the other side* of change? Once you made it through a meaningful change, I would hazard a guess that in retrospection, it was rather beautiful, or at least purposeful, to cross the change bridge.

We increase our comfort with discomfort *through* discomfort, and the process doesn't have to be as rocky as some might think. No one wants to be uncomfortable all the time, and in any big change, the reality is that we truly aren't uncomfortable forever. Courageous change leads to time-limited discomfort (grappling). A flare in emotions won't be the predominant norm for any incident. It is often *incidental and fleeting* ... The more comfortable you become with this idea, the easier it is to have a challenging dialogue for the sake of change. What we seek to gain from this work is far more beautiful than the trepidation that we initially feel.

As I continued to reflect on my frustration with cowardly leaders who had power and influence but refused to use it when a matter of equity/inequity would require it, I characterized cowardice as inaction including silence (not in introspection, but for the long term). They wouldn't *say* what needed to be said. They wouldn't *do* what needed to be done. Amid my disappointment with stagnant leaders, I started investigating the concept of risk-taking and what contributes to leaders being risk averse.

In my reflecting on the work of Margie Warrell, I use the image of a bungee jumper to represent a leader who exaggerates the likelihood that something will go wrong. Although the likelihood that the cord will break is minuscule, I'm not sure I ever want to try bungee jumping and take the chance that it *might*. We often exaggerate the likelihood that the dialogue about inequities and racism will be disastrous—or will it? Will it go wrong? Well, it probably won't be a catastrophe, but in all truth the tough conversations might go poorly. That brings me to the next stage of my imagining ...

Envision an elephant on a tightrope. The likelihood that this elephant will fall off that rope is pretty high, but the consequences of what will happen if he falls might, again, not be as disastrous as feared. There might be a big, deep lake below him or thick, deep brush that will catch him, and this elephant will be fine! Similarly, the equity conversation may go poorly, but perhaps not as poorly as you fear. And even if it does go wrong, things may occur that mediate the negative outcome, like that lake or brush below the elephant.

Let's be realistic: equity engagement can be precarious, and a number of unanticipated negative outcomes may occur. In other words, it may go badly. But, moving to my next imagination, the likelihood is that you can handle it. Imagine you are hang gliding and a wind gust takes you off course. The urgency of the moment will kick in, and you do what is necessary. I have experienced this in tough race-based dialogues. My heart may be beating faster and my breathing turns more shallow, but I know that I can lean into the outcome.

All these images are vital considerations; the likelihood that it will go badly is probably less than you think. If it does go badly, the consequences may not be as disastrous as you fear. Still, if something hard happens, you can handle it (I promise you!). These three images—the bungee jumper, the elephant on the tightrope, and the hang glider—are focused on you as a leader. Perceived risk in the realm of equity provides Mirror Moments that challenge us to leverage our reactions.

This section began with a quote from Margie Warrell, who has a lot of incredible things to teach us about risk. One of her points is fundamental for equity leaders. It elevates our thinking to the impact of our actions on the circumstances around us—encouraging us to consider the *impact of inaction*. Doing nothing is doing something! And doing nothing is not an acceptable option as we advance equity. Our field and even our families are impacted by our actions or our inaction. Our spheres of influence as leaders are significant, as we're serving in an era that implores us to do and say more.

The imagery of inaction. Here we go: Imagine, finally, a large turtle crossing a road. I have actually come across this before. The turtle was making good progress as I drove around him, avoiding hitting him. But when my trip took me back to that same street heading in the opposite direction, I noticed that the turtle seemed to have just stopped moving. It was as if the turtle thought, *I changed my mind about crossing this street*, or *I think I'm good right here after all*.

Yes, there's tremendous risk in his attempt, but imagine what's on the other side of his courageous choice if only he followed through! We must keep striving—bungee-cording, tightrope walking, hang gliding, and yes, crossing all the way to the other side of the street. Human fear impedes courageous change. So when any risk feels threatening, check in with yourself. Are you overestimating the probability that something will go wrong or exaggerating the consequences? Are you underestimating your ability to handle the repercussions? Or are you stuck in the status quo and not considering the cost of inaction?

When you envision the goal, it allows you to push through risk to get to the other side. Ultimately, courage is required for change, and committing to tough equity leadership actions is accompanied by *grace* to carry out that commitment to change. We are not simply doing this work for the sake of doing it. We're not merely changing things for the sake of changing them—we are disrupting the status quo for the sake of assuring the conditions for equity to evolve and grow with its impact remaining for future generations. Change is an act of courage and, ultimately, an act of joy.

TAKE THE CHANCE—UPDATE THIS OLD HOUSE!

> *So have no fear of them, for nothing is covered that will not be revealed, or hidden that will not be known.*
>
> —MATTHEW 10:26

Change-averse people fein comfort; "We got it. This has worked fine for years. Why do we need to change it?" Well, because people are different now—times are different. Or perhaps it is because times *haven't* changed! The causes of inequities in our society have remained unaddressed. Many of our efforts are a demonstration of the old adage of putting lipstick on a pig. Everything around us may appear different, except for our practices. It's comfortable to rely on what has worked for a long time. Yes, that old protocol might be comfortable for you, but consider who it's *not* comfortable for. Who knows, once we change that practice, maybe you'll discover it wasn't optimal for *you* either. We often fail to see or take into account the benefit—the necessity—of progressing.

To offer a more lighthearted example: as an HGTV fan (perhaps the sociologist in me), I'm always fascinated by the moment when something appears outdated. There's an interval of time when a car might be five years old but it still looks like a new car. Then, all of a sudden, the car looks out of style. A kitchen looks contemporary for years and years, and instantly it becomes old news: wrong colors, wrong styles. The same goes for clothing. "I've worn this suit, it still fits, and it's timeless"—until the lapel cut is wrong or the tie is too wide.

My team once used an instructional video about servant leadership in an orientation that took place twice a year. The video message was powerful, clear, and motivating, but I vividly recall the moment when we pulled it up and it suddenly seemed dated. The offices that were shown seemed from another era, the clothing was clearly from a long-past decade, and the hairstyles ... Well, suffice it to say that fashion had moved to another place! The trappings of the video became a huge distraction to the important content that was being shared. The lipstick on that pig was obviously wearing off.

We are tempted—in so many facets of culture—to think that things are good and that all this talk about diversity is just making matters worse. As the director of our local health department and beginning all-staff work on health equity and social justice, I received a staff complaint that said, "We didn't have these problems with race until you made us start talking about all this." Hmmm ... All too many feel that the old tried-and-true has been working for so long, so let's just leave things alone and live our lives. No, we need to grapple and grow ...

Circumstances are changing all around us in public health and the world in general. Tragically, they seem to be changing for the worse. People are getting sicker, life expectancy has declined, more babies are dying, and no one can deny the disturbing patterns surrounding gun violence in our country. What a profound opportunity to ask ourselves as leaders, "Are we out of date? Do we need to do something completely different?" The spirit of equity leadership cries out, "Enough is enough! We need a complete overhaul of this house!" I don't mean a little paint and changing the cabinet hardware but a refurbishment where you walk in and don't even recognize the place. We must change ...

In my basement, I still have a phone jack for a landline. I could insist that someone use my phone jack simply because it works and I happen to have a telephone in addition to my cell phone. That person (likely my son, who I refuse to let throw away my old phone) would likely wonder, "Why on earth do we still have this?" So, yes, the phone jack still functions, but why would anyone bother when we have better, more efficient ways of communicating? And why is it so difficult for me to discard the old phone and stop paying the bundle fee for the landline?!

Fellow equity leaders—unplug your landlines and move forward. While you're at it, don't just put that old phone away but refurbish everything so that the landline jack is removed and no longer presents a

> **FOR THOSE TIRED OF TALKING ABOUT EQUITY, THE IRONY IS THAT THE MORE WE TALK ABOUT IT, THE LESS WE WILL NEED TO TALK ABOUT IT.**

temptation to backtrack (I promise to do this with my phone jack soon!). What are the remnants of the past in our society that keep us from moving forward toward equity? The security blankets of the past that keep us stuck—what are the items and memories that we continue to personally hold on to that impede change?

For those tired of talking about equity, the irony is that the more we talk about it, the less we will need to talk about it. Doing the heavy work *first* brings the change that will make equity practices second nature. Well, we take three steps forward and two steps back—there is progress but also retraction. Why allow the bait to regress to an old way of doing things? We typically have a short attention span and want to move on to the next thing, except when it comes to equity matters. So let's be true to that tendency and all move on *while* bringing equity with us.

COURAGEOUSLY STEPPING OFF THE EQUALITY BANDWAGON

One day our descendants will think it incredible that we paid so much attention to things like the amount of melanin in our skin or the shape of our eyes or our gender instead of the unique identities of each of us as complex human beings.

— FRANKLIN THOMAS

The 2020 murder of George Floyd resurrected a season of unrest filled with demonstrations, disruption, and dialogue. It also illuminated the dire need for equity leaders who could guide change and transformation. A common response among corporations and various organizations was the creation of positions that held titles like "VP of equity" and "director of DEI." In most cases, these positions were created without staff, budget, or broad organizational support. Very few seemed to consider critical questions such as "How will we assure that equity positions are integrated and valued across the company?"

As it turned out, this intention didn't come to fruition. Companies seemingly did not ask important questions or even follow through. They put words on paper to describe a role (again, getting credit without doing the work). So what happened as soon as the budget turned or the grant ended? The equity positions in many cases were the first to go. This same pattern is ubiquitous—a problem I see in continuous waves. Maybe *you* were hired to check a box. If so, then you understand the frustration. But you are still where you are for the purpose of advancing change, to push us ahead, and to—at the very least—make people uncomfortable and challenge the status quo. We can tell if we fail to lean into courageous change when there is a sentiment of relief in the atmosphere with others thinking, *Phew. Thank goodness that wasn't as bad as I thought it would be!* No one grappled. No one changed. And everyone missed an opportunity to experience the growth that change brings—the necessity and reality of courageous change.

Our country is continuously driven by an *equality* model (I keep telling you so that you'll never let this realization disappear). It is baked into our democracy. Equality means sameness: we strive to treat everyone the same. *"We hold these truths to be self-evident that all men are created equal."* Rarely do we allow ourselves to reflect on the context of that statement and who was excluded, who made that statement, and what their intentions were. Case in point: the US golden rule challenges us to treat people like we want to be treated. This results in people being treated the same and, even worse, centering their own wants rather than the wants of others. Nevertheless, the notion of equality is a cultural bedrock.

The model of equity leadership tasks us with applying an abundance of courage to move and, instead of centering ourselves, to center and assess the needs of those we seek to serve, those individuals likely who have needs and wants different from our own. I often find myself pausing before making a key decision. I have to be intentional to assess whether I am falling into an equality frame because the socializing is so deep. My thought process requires me to slow down my decision-making to reflect on whether I am acting through an *equality*-driven narrative. Getting off autopilot requires that we think differently ...

I invite you to retrain your brain. It is preprogrammed for equality. How we approach any situation, any given day, allows us the opportunity to build our *equity* acumen. What we fear most is fleeting, but what we seek to gain will forever change this world. Have courage! The world needs you.

LEARNING LESSONS: THE COURAGEOUS CHANGE

- Saying the word *equity* doesn't mean that we are *doing* equity.
- Equity leadership is for all, not just BIPOC folx.
- We are all risk averse. Building courage muscles makes us risk *reverse*!
- Overcoming resistance requires us to overcome hesitance.

MIRROR MOMENTS: THE COURAGEOUS CHANGE

1. What was the last courageous moment you had—big or small? What did it feel like? What was the aftermath of your actions?
2. Think about a leader who has inspired you. What qualities were you moved by? Also, consider one who frustrated and enervated you. Reflect upon the differences in these two leaders.
3. At an institutional level (not an interpersonal level), describe a time when you were a change agent (i.e., when your actions improved a situation or resolved a problem). What feelings did you experience in deciding to act? What feelings did you experience after the action?

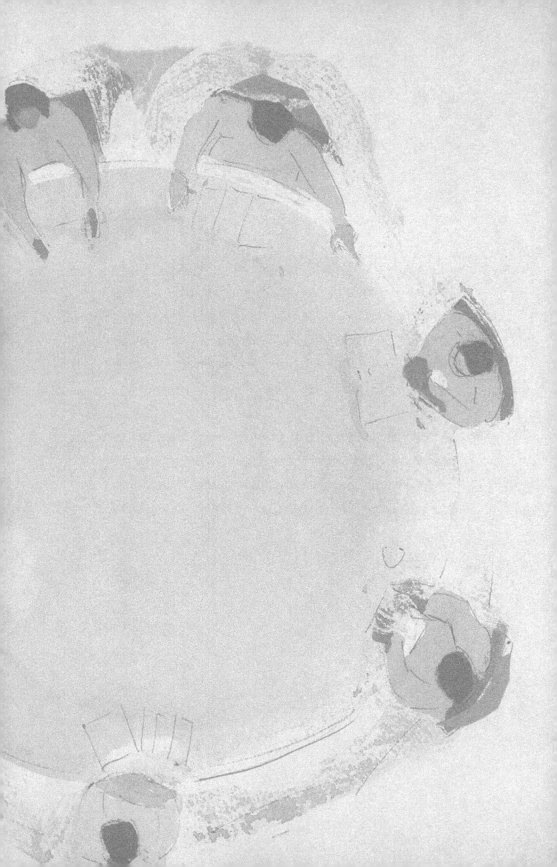

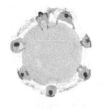

CHAPTER NINE

WHEN TRUTH AND FACTS COLLIDE

*When I was a child, I talked like a child, I thought
like a child, I reasoned like a child. When I became a
man, I put the ways of childhood behind me.*

—1 CORINTHIANS 13:11

T here will be some grappling in this chapter. There will be reflection, storytelling, outrage, confusion, and sadness. It all fits in the equity lens.

I once spoke at a conference where the theme was "narrative change," and I titled my keynote address "Storytelling and Telling Stories: Truth, Lies, and the Narratives We Build." As I reflected on the importance of community voice and storytelling as powerful tools in that regard, I was reminded of the play on words from my childhood. Growing up, we weren't allowed to say *you're a liar*. That was considered rude and unkind. We got in a lot of trouble for using the *L*-word. So instead of telling someone that they were a liar, we would say, "You're *telling a story*," usually prefaced with a long, tantalizing "Oooooooooo!"

This tension between the realities of telling a story and the truths of storytelling elevate the need for authenticity. Are we being transparent and trustworthy, or are we constructing a narrative to meet our ends? In my childhood paradigm, if you said that somebody was telling a story, then you couldn't accept their words as truth. They were making something up. They were fibbing! Just as *telling a story* stifles truth or positions a false narrative, on the flip side storytelling invites truth and elevates lived experiences—vital ingredients in equity leadership.

Our challenge as equity leaders is to allow the lived experiences of others to resonate as truth instead of saying, "Well, I don't think it actually happened that way," or "I don't think they meant it that way." How can we be authentic and hear what we might be opposed to hearing or see what we might be opposed to seeing? Before you assume that someone is telling a story, listen to their storytelling.

STORYTELLING—A GLIMPSE INTO ANOTHER'S LIVED EXPERIENCE

*Many stories matter. Stories have been used to dispossess
and to malign. But stories can also be used to empower,
and to humanize. Stories can break the dignity of a people.
But stories can also repair that broken dignity.*

—CHIMAMANDA NGOZI ADICHIE

The timing of this chapter coincided with a number of pivotal events in our nation. *Roe v. Wade* had just been overturned, and I had to reflect on the question "What is this leadership moment?" The leadership moment began to reveal itself further as several other incidents coalesced. One key incident occurred when I learned that my research was cited in Chief Justice John Roberts's response to the Supreme Court decision on *Roe v. Wade*.[8] When I first received a text message from a staff member sharing this fact with me, my reaction was confusion. *That can't be true*, I said to myself.

The moment was conflicting. At first, I didn't know the details, and my coauthors and colleagues were also shocked by this fact. Our cited publication presented a finding that described that most women recognize that they are pregnant by fifteen weeks of gestation. Justice Roberts's position stated, "That line (in the document seeking to terminate *Roe v. Wade*) never made sense. A woman's right to abortion should extend far enough to ensure a reasonable opportunity to choose." He used our research findings, affirming that fifteen weeks were justifiable to seek the middle ground in a divisive issue. So, *deep breath* … and let the grappling begin.

I have always posited that the choices people make are determined by the choices that people have. Limiting choices in general rarely leads to the best outcomes. As such, in a play on words, I would describe myself as *pro-choices*, simply because the goal isn't to narrow people's options, but rather to *expand* the options available. On the other end of this grappling spectrum, let's move from considering *pro-choices* to the pro-life discourse … I believe that life begins in utero, and I also believe that life is much more than birth. If we are concerned about life, we must be concerned about life in utero and life after delivery. A review of infant mortality data reveals that a large and disproportionate number of infants who die before they reach the age of one year is due to the complications of the *context* of their births and their mother's pregnancy.

---

8   Katie Yoder, "Why Did Chief Justice Roberts Disagree with Overturning *Roe v. Wade?*" *National Catholic Register*, June 26, 2022, https://www.ncregister.com/cna/why-did-chief-justice-roberts-disagree-with-overturning-roe-v-wade.

As such, the opposite corollary to the *pro-life* frame is what I would further describe as *pro-life-course*. A life-course orientation requires us to be concerned about children from the point they are conceived through adulthood. We must care about the well-being of children as infants in their homes, as toddlers, and beyond in their schools. Pro-life-course aligns with pro-choices, offering a shifted, more inclusive narrative.

The divisive nature of the debate across varied and diverse groups after the overturning of Roe v. Wade *provided a very complicated dialogue, void of civility and seemingly full of people telling stories without inviting the storytelling of the people most affected by the decision.* It is symptomatic of how poorly we communicate across *difference* and *disagreement*. So I ask, *What could leadership look like in a moment like this?* Equity leadership seeks to look and truly *see* the circumstances—the evidence and facts and how these align with people's lives.

THE DIVISIVE NATURE OF THE DEBATE ACROSS VARIED AND DIVERSE GROUPS AFTER THE OVERTURNING OF *ROE V. WADE* PROVIDED A VERY COMPLICATED DIALOGUE, VOID OF CIVILITY AND SEEMINGLY FULL OF PEOPLE TELLING STORIES WITHOUT INVITING THE STORYTELLING OF THE PEOPLE MOST AFFECTED BY THE DECISION.

Having your scholarly work cited by a Supreme Court justice should be a moment of pride, but in this case, it was also a moment of conflict. Allow me to share a few truths in my life that directly affected my response to this situation. Some storytelling …

Mamie J. Knight was my grandmother, whom I have mentioned earlier. We lovingly called her "Grandtie," and she was a woman of great resilience and strength. She was also the poster child for a common saying in the African American church: "I don't look like what I've been through." Grandtie was full of joy, laughter, and purpose. A few weeks before she passed away at the age of ninety-five, she called me into her room and said, "I need to tell you something, and I don't want you to speak a word of this to anybody until I'm gone."

She shared that Sam White (known to be my grandfather) was not, in fact, my grandfather. In other words, Sam White was not my mother's father. I have to admit, I wasn't surprised at all by this information because my grandmother's complexion was very fair, as was my mother's. Sam White, on the other hand, was a dark Black man. I always thought to myself, *Man, those genes didn't merge at all!* You would think that my mother wouldn't be an amalgamation of both skin colors. My mother's complexion was so fair that Grandtie frequently admonished her to go outside and get some sun!

So learning that Sam White was not my mother's biological father made sense. Grandtie then proceeded to tell me her story about walking home from work one day and being pushed into the bushes by a young white man. She had been raped and assaulted that day. My mother was the product of that assault. The facts of my lineage—my heritage—merged into the truth of that awful, racialized incident.

As I listened to my grandmother's horrid story, I was overwhelmed by silence. I simply and deeply listened. I knew that Grandtie was one of thirteen children in her family. She continued her story by saying, "White folks really liked my daddy. They would give him hand-me-down clothes and extra food to help him provide for all of us." As she continued, what emerged was the answer to my unspoken questions: *What did you do? How did you "decide" what to do after this terrible assault?*

As a family, they had a choice to make, but did they really? They knew who the assailant was, and my grandmother Mamie and her parents had to decide how to handle the situation. Grandtie and her family chose silence ... Again, the choices people make are determined by the choices they *have. What were the choices they had? How is executing choice an act of power, even in the absence of ideal choices?* And so, she gave birth to my mother—my lifeblood—in a moment that could be described as both pro-choice and pro-life. It was also a moment where the truth of the potential consequences collided with the facts of an assault.

Equity leaders are often faced with moments of of contradictory choice—to speak or remain silent—to cry loud or hunker down—all of which, as in Grandtie's experience, carry consequences. In my grandmother's case, the question was not simply what choice did she have and what choice did she make, but also what choices *did she really* have and what choices *could* she actually make. The conditions of equity similarly are not straightforward or easy to draw conclusions from.

As I reflect on these critical life events, I can imagine the innocent responses to my sharing with others the fact that "my research was cited by the Supreme Court." I can't help but hear that childhood retort, "Oooooo, you tellin' a story!" or sharing that my mother was conceived as a result of a racist attack. Again, "Oooooo, you tellin' a story." But no, I'm not telling a story. I'm sharing a moment of my own storytelling with you. Increasing our comfort with our own stories—even if unexpected, as was the case in my origin story—helps shine a light on the truth and facts of our lives and the potential they have to collide and contradict each other. Truth is more clearly illuminated through stories, lived experiences, and even qualitative data.

How do our truths reconcile themselves on our journeys and contribute to our being the leaders that we are? The fact that my staff was up at nine o'clock on a Friday night reading the Supreme Court decision was baffling to me. First of all, who actually reads decisions of the SCOTUS, and second, why wasn't my staff out at the movies enjoying themselves or relaxing after a long week? Instead, they texted me with a screenshot of the startling citation from my research paper. There I was, "R. Canady," cited in a document responding to the inevitable dismissal of *Roe v. Wade*—someone who desperately seeks to find the middle ground and stands as a peacemaker and reconciler and also one whose personal heritage is the direct consequence of a mother's unimaginable choice.

We can't escape the truth of doing what is *needed*, whether courage compels us or cowardice threatens to get in the way. If the narrative of pro-life-course and pro-choices helps advance *dialogue*, reconciles those in opposition, or pushes us to think more deeply, then we have progressed. When facing such challenging dialogues, we must avoid a natural tendency to shut down. Perhaps you can relate: "This is where I am, and I'm not talking to anyone who doesn't share this point of view because I don't want to be convinced, persuaded, or otherwise informed."

Truth manifests in many different ways in the lives of those we serve as equity leaders. Have the dialogue and listen to the stories told …

TRUTH, FACTS, AND MISINTERPRETATION

There's a world of difference between truth and
facts. Facts can obscure the truth.

—MAYA ANGELOU

Sometimes the same words tell a completely different story to the speaker and the hearer. I recall serving as a mentor for a national health equity fellowship. We held a retreat at a *remote* retreat center. Having caught a late flight, and riding for what seemed like forever (going literally over the river and through the woods), we finally arrived at our destination. The hostess greeted us warmly and let me know that they had reserved a private room for me as opposed to the common sleeping areas that the fellows shared. As we walked outside the welcome center, where most of the other fellows and staff were staying, and *rounded the bend*, we arrived at an isolated room that faced the woods.

I commented with a bit of trepidation, "Wow, I could scream at the top of my lungs back here and no one would hear me!" Her gleeful reply was "Oh, yes! Just scream to your heart's content. Let it all out!"

ARE YOU SAYING WHAT YOU MEAN AND MEANING WHAT YOU SAY IN WAYS THAT ARE UNDERSTOOD AS YOU INTENDED?

This episode has become an iconic incident among the fellowship staff and cohorts. That kind lady didn't catch my drift … The situation brings up a great question for all of us: *Are you saying what you mean and meaning what you say in ways that are understood as you intended?* The facts relayed by the hostess (yes, no one will hear you yell) were a complete contradiction to my truths in that instance (I'm feeling unsafe in the isolated room). The onus lies with us as equity leaders to speak, vet, affirm, and repeat. Indeed, we see and hear things not as they are but as *we* are.

Another occurrence involves the birth of my firstborn son, Mark Howard, at twenty-eight weeks' gestation. While attending a routine prenatal visit, I was informed that my blood pressure was alarmingly high and I was being sent right over to the hospital. I was instructed not to go home, not to pack a bag—they would take care of things. The goal of my hospital admission was to delay a premature delivery. The plan was to put me on bedrest on my left side and to treat me with steroids to help the baby's lungs mature quickly, just in case delivery could not be prevented.

A couple of days into my admission, I was awakened one morning by the appearance of a gurney in my room, accompanied by a parade of providers. I was told that I was being prepped for an emergency C-section. Understandably startled, I asked, "Wait a minute! Can we talk about this? Is somebody going to talk to me and explain what is going on?" The answer that I received was that they had already spoken to my husband and that we needed to proceed quickly. My obstetrician arrived and "reassuringly" said, "Don't you worry about a thing; you will be fine." That *I am going to be fine* is not at all the point in the moment! Somehow, this did not seem like the right time to resist or take a stand on principle. But the facts that prompted their sudden intervention did not consider my truths as the patient. Once again, silence became the action of choice in this moment of truth.

About five months into his all-too-short life of six months, Howard was moved from the NICU (neonatal intensive care unit) to the PICU (pediatric intensive care unit). The prior goal of the neo-natologists had been to "get this baby breathing room air" (in other words, get him off the ventilator). In their minds, if Howard remained on a vent, not breathing room air without mechanical assistance, they were not succeeding.

On the other hand, the priority of the ped intensivists was weight gain for my beautiful son, and as such, their recommendation was this: "Let's 'trach' this kid." A tracheotomy would assist Howard's breathing and lower the calories expended to breathe, thus contributing to weight gain. Getting him fatter and healthier was a key metric of their success. Were either of these approaches wrong? Were the strategies and recommendations based on facts? Somewhere amid these two perspectives was my somewhat overlooked *truth* as a loving (and often desperate, in this situation) parent.

Whose truths prevail? Whose needs are centered, and whose story is being told? The stories that my son and I lived through in the sick-care system (yes, the healthcare system is more accurately described as the sick-care system) were numerous. The team (however grateful for them I was) did not center the voice of the one most affected by the problem at hand—Howard and his parents. *Who was marginalized? Whose facts prevailed, and whose truths were negated? And how does the failure to consider truths contribute to misinterpretation?*

A final story offers a response to those questions. After Howard died, I realized that all our pictures of him had his nasal cannula in the photo or an IV taped to him. I asked a friend, who is an exceptional and gifted artist, "Can you do a portrait of Howard without the medical equipment?" The artist enthusiastically obliged. Upon completion of the portrait, we had a big reveal! My artist friend was beaming. "I want to watch you as you look at the picture for the first time." "Okay!" I enthusiastically responded, eager to see the true Howard. So he positioned me and unveiled the portrait. My face immediately fell. The artist knew what had happened inside me and felt so bad! "I missed it. I missed it! I'll take it back. Talk to me about what you're seeing and I'll revise it."

WHO WAS MARGINALIZED? WHOSE FACTS PREVAILED, AND WHOSE TRUTHS WERE NEGATED? AND HOW DOES THE FAILURE TO CONSIDER TRUTHS CONTRIBUTE TO MISINTERPRETATION?

What I realized at that moment was that he would never be able to see what I saw in my precious baby—my small, dear, adorable warrior child. He saw the fighter, but the warrior was a sick infant. Years later, as I look at my pictures of Howard, I realize how accurate the artist's depiction was, but the truth is that my unbounded love only saw the glint in his eye, the soft half smile, and the small yet chubby cheeks. Yes, I could step back and see how sick Howard looked in actuality … but he was an adorable angel in the eyes of his mother. Indeed, we do see things as *we* are. I saw Howard through the eyes of a mother—breathing, hoping, expecting, fingers crossed, and prayers up. The artist friend saw a more realistic fact-based image that misinterpreted the truth of who Howard was, and *is*, to me.

WELL-MEANING VERSUS WELL-DOING

And let us not grow weary of doing good, for in due season we will reap, if we do not give up.

—GALATIANS 6:9

Socialization can also contribute to our personal and collective misinterpretations. Let's go back to the earlier point about the golden rule, a common social principle in our society. "Do unto others as you would have others do unto you," or "treat people the way you want to be treated." It sounds good at face value, but placing ourselves as the gold standard for how to treat others is fraught with challenges.

Take, for example, something as simple as using the elevator or the stairs. If you are a fitness-focused step counter, you likely want to take the steps. If you assume others feel the same, you discount the needs of another who may have a physical condition (seen or unseen) that impairs their ability to use the stairs, or they may just not like taking stairs. The risks are much higher when addressing more weighty matters such as our social identities. But looking at the intent of that phrase that we call the golden rule, our challenge of applying it can be unpacked with that little word *as* … Do unto others *as* you would have them do unto you.

Most people associate the word *as* with *similarly*. But others do not want to be treated similarly to you. Your needs will be different from the needs of others, and vice versa. Rather, the goal is to treat others like *they* want to be treated, not similar to how *you* want to be treated or replicated in terms of what you would want done to/for you. While this may seem to be splitting hairs, it is a common source of angst and frustration in our society. Meeting people at the point of their needs (rather than at the point of your needs) will guide us to authentic and effective engagement as equity leaders. (In the spirit of avoiding misinterpretation, let me share this: Although the golden rule applies a Judeo-Christian principle, it is not a biblical quote/verse.)

I hope that the stories in this chapter have ignited the affective leadership side of who you are and even spurred you to think about your own lived experiences that have shaped your worldview. Many emotionally powerful life moments are draped in conflict or misinterpretation. In a conversation I had with a member of our communications staff after the realization that my work was cited in the *Roe v. Wade* decision, I admitted that "I'm still grappling with that fact. The truth is, I don't know what to say or how to say it." They suggested that people want to hear from me and know what I'm thinking, but I simply did not know what to say (thank you, self-awareness, for making that realization okay). That's the leadership tension. In response to my grappling, my communications colleague asked, "Don't you think you can set aside the very personal event in your life with your grandmother? Can't you just say something as the CEO?" *But how would one do that?*

Tension in leadership—especially equity leadership—and tension in the *facts versus the lived experience* must be allowed space to exist. If the SCOTUS *Roe v. Wade* opinion offers any opportunity, I'd say that it is to set a table that is bigger and wider. It calls for broader dialogue and more inclusive language across our differences. *Resist the temptation to narrow the table, limit the seats at the table, or leave the table.* Make space so that if you don't want to sit right next to me because of a disagreement, then you can sit across the table so you can subtly learn from the opinion of someone different from you.

> **RESIST THE TEMPTATION TO NARROW THE TABLE, LIMIT THE SEATS AT THE TABLE, OR LEAVE THE TABLE.**

Hear, *learn*, and *think*. I have used story-telling as the technique to share some of my truths. What are your truths? What are your stories? Sometimes facts and truth simply collide. They may not even reconcile but they may connect parallel journeys. As equity leaders, we must recognize these moments and realize that they can be leveraged for our greatest demonstration of leadership. Show up fully while keeping your ears, eyes, mind, and heart open to everyone else.

LEARNING LESSONS: WHEN TRUTH AND FACTS COLLIDE

- Your lived experiences shape how you experience world events.
- Stories filled with truths can be more powerful than facts.
- Seek to shift from well-meaning to well-*doing*.
- Treat people as *they* would like to be treated.

MIRROR MOMENTS: WHEN TRUTH AND FACTS COLLIDE

1. Consider a time when you experienced an important shift in your understanding of what was true. This could be a personal awakening or an awakening to the true nature of a process, a job, or a way of thinking. It could also be a broad cultural shift that many others experienced as well. Try to identify a moment when things, as they were, changed for you significantly.

2. When has your personal story been discounted? In other words, when has your narrative been taken from you? What in that experience can be used to ensure that you do not replicate such actions with others?

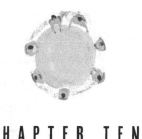

CHAPTER TEN

CONTINUATION OVER CONCLUSION

To succeed, jump as quickly at opportunities as you do at conclusions.

—BENJAMIN FRANKLIN

I had the privilege of vacationing in Belize to celebrate my birthday. Toward the end of my trip, while riding in a golf cart (the motorized vehicle of choice in Belize), I had an unexpected sign encounter as we approached an intersection. The stop sign seemed very familiar—octagonal in shape, block letters as expected, and positioned at a similar height to what I was accustomed. After taking a second look, my surprise turned to wonder and curiosity. The sign was green instead of red …

While my mind continued to reflect on the apparent contradiction, my heart was energized by the symbolic significance. Like this sign, there are many social indicators that tell us to stop in our forward-moving equity work, but in the face of those messages, we must seek the subliminal and direct callings that encourage us to continue on.

The shape tells me to stop, the color tells me to go, and my forward momentum leads me to continue even as I experience counterintuitive messages or those that I have never before encountered.

We are socialized, trained, and taught to seek the conclusion—the outcome—of our actions. Think about that kid in the back seat asking, "Are we there yet?" Leaders have the natural inclination to ask this time-honored road trip question. More intellectually, I have heard it articulated as "How will we know our actions have been effective? What metrics will we use to evaluate our equity intervention?" There are many evaluation scientists working on that question, but I would submit that the childhood "Are we there yet?" puts us in a mindset to forgo considering the value of the equity journey. *Equity as a journey—not simply a destination—allows us to focus on the systems and processes that currently contribute to the negative outcomes that all too many people experience.* As equity leaders, we are also focused on the *process* of health equity. Ours is an ongoing action of staying the course and building momentum for change.

> EQUITY AS A JOURNEY—NOT SIMPLY A DESTINATION—ALLOWS US TO FOCUS ON THE SYSTEMS AND PROCESSES THAT CURRENTLY CONTRIBUTE TO THE NEGATIVE OUTCOMES THAT ALL TOO MANY PEOPLE EXPERIENCE.

There is an unexpected irony in what we do. If things unfold in ways that feel natural and familiar, then we are likely not operating at a level of deep equity. Disruptive and innovative thinking, as is needed in this space, is uncomfortable and awkward. It is counterintuitive. It fits but doesn't quite fit. It is the "square peg in a round hole," but more accurately, it is the round peg in a square hole. It *will* fit, but not precisely until we see systems adapting. We must continually check our complacency. The hallmark of equity momentum is the continuous and iterative nature of our efforts, undaunted by the impostor syndrome that is sure to follow along with us.

Think of the situated-ness of our work and responsibilities. For those of us reading this book now, we are situated in the *now* of our current events; our strategies and resources are different from those that paved the way for our action historically. For those reading this book, or a similar treatise, *years from now*, the battles and victories should be different, especially if we did our work well in this generation. The effort continues, but it evolves to meet the next context and needs. We are leaders *at* this time and *for* this time. Our goals and methods are contextualized by what's happening around us.

My thinking continues to shift. I believe in incremental change, but this does not mean slow and plodding. There is an urgency pushing us to be intentional and focused. Think about the quality-improvement model Plan/Do/Study/Act (PDSA). In public health, we also accelerate that model with rapid PDSA. Just because we are focused on the process does not mean that moving forward with intent and pace is overlooked. As leaders, we are the cadence keepers of our equity strategies. When we apply the image of baby steps, it is usually an admonition to take small sets—go little by little. But I have reframed my mindset about baby steps. Having spent a significant amount of time with a toddler, I realized that baby steps may be small, but toddlers can fly! You may have seen a mother running after a baby-stepping toddler who scurried away rapidly with glee! As a result, I have shifted from being an incrementalist to a *rapid incrementalist* and have seen the paradigm work in public health practice.

The process of continuation is not formulaic and transactional—advancing equity is rarely routine. In rapid incrementalism, as with rapid PDSA, you plan for something, do it, and then review what you did—asking yourself how it turned out. From those results, you tweak and act again. It is not only a continuous cycle, but it is a *praxis*. Paulo Freire defines praxis as reflection plus action. Think about what you are going to do, do it, and then reflect on it again as you continually move forward.

The Mirror Moments are designed to build your comfort with reflection and introspection as you cultivate an equity leadership philosophy and praxis. This *process* keeps us from becoming stagnant. In evaluation science, process outcomes are as important as the terminal outcomes. As an equity leader, I observe process outcomes such as increasing trust among community members or trust among staff. These combined with relationship building all contribute to the process outcome of social capital, which is then leveraged to keep us continuing and advancing the work. There is an end in sight, but we only arrive through the journey and continuation.

When are the times and circumstances ready for us to put our foot on the gas and speed up? When do the circumstances mandate that we slow down? People often complain that we're taking two steps forward and three steps back, thinking it a waste of effort. But movement is movement, whether we're moving forward or backward. Three steps back can give you a different vantage point and perspective, especially having seen two steps ahead—we now have different intel than before that informs our next steps forward, making it more strategic and effective. You gain insight and become sensitive to the systems in place that impede progress.

Keep asking the questions! Is this a time when you can push? You might feel it is now the time to drive people forward—or *pull* them forward, if you must. You know that moment when you are all linking arms and moving ahead, but you also understand that there will be times when issues of psychological safety (for your team, the community, or other partners) will prompt you to slow down. We remain on the journey, understanding that the pace will ebb, flow, and even accelerate.

Incrementalism as praxis looks like this: "We planned and engaged with the community, but now let's do some reflection on how it went—what were the challenges, and what went well along the way? There will be things to tweak, and then we can continue to partner with the community." The time you take to assess is time spent moving forward, and in many ways, leveraging those steps back results in powerful momentum.

TAKE YOUR TIME AND HURRY UP—GO FAST, SLOW DOWN, AND ADVANCE

I have been impressed with the urgency of doing. Knowing is not enough; we must apply. Being willing is not enough; we must do.

—LEONARDO DA VINCI

I continue to encourage you to strengthen your equity leadership skill of recognizing contradictions and the counterintuitive. We might expect to read/hear, "Take your time but hurry up." That small conjunction "but" can flip trust and relationship on its head. By saying *but* in that phrase, aren't you actually telling me to not take my time? Remember, as equity leaders we are saying what we mean and meaning what we say.

Moving this work forward and sensing the right time to do so requires you to assess what others need and *observe* what's happening around you. Your *instincts* alone may require unlearning and relearning to clear out old practices and bad habits. How can you be an adaptive leader who shifts while feeling out that pace and cadence? Giving yourself permission to take your time and hurry up is a first step. Equity leaders do seemingly contradictory things. Taking your time does not mean *slowing down*. In this context, it means taking the gift of time assigned to you to do something with it as a leader.

Let's find a better iteration of *but*. If you are an early adopter of equity principles, you will often find yourself *leading up*. I describe this as the "Excuse me, but …" phenomenon. It starts as an ever-so-gentle nudge, ping, or even a figurative pinch! *Excuse me, but have we ever considered … Excuse me, but this seems to overlook … Excuse me, but we have to talk about this!* It is a technique that shifts the dialogue toward equity, especially when you see an opportunity to do so being bypassed.

I sometimes would ask myself, *Why isn't someone else saying what needs to be said?* Being the "Excuse me, but …" (for brevity, let's call it *EMB*) person seems lonely. Trust me, it almost feels like Sisyphus pushing his boulder up the mountain. And then there is the risk of being typecast as the EMB. I can recall being in numerous meetings where people were agreeing to several decisions contrary to equity or, at best, did not *consider* equity. It seemed they were agreeing to these points, knowing that I would eventually ride in on my equity bandwagon. People assumed that we'd pause because Renée (the EMB) would say what she always *has* to say about equity. If this kind of pressure intimidates you—and it *is* very intimidating—I encourage you to take heart.

I have seen the shift in three separate organizations where I eventually moved from the EMB role to more of a concurring "amen corner" role! In my silence—which is a powerful place to be—I observed as others raised the equity banner I had previously held up in isolation. Once your team internalizes equity principles, then they can speak up and you can offer support. That is when you know people are getting on the same page … *It is a gratifying feeling when you observe someone else address the inequity red flags that contradict equity goals. I get the satisfaction of sitting back and smiling, saying to myself, "That's exactly what I was thinking."*

Take your time judiciously, swiftly, and intentionally! Doing the extra work on the front end makes the journey much easier. This isn't about taking *more* time but rather shifting the time or using the time differently. Rushing will take up more of my time when I've got to go back and fix the oversights in what went too fast. Slow down so that people understand, are invested, and can have input or improve upon the decisions affecting them. That is why pacing the dialogue with an EMB prompt can be beneficial.

Listen, there *is* beauty in baby steps, but this process is also much more fluid and nuanced. Equity decision-making and equity action are not linear. Looking back and assessing where you came from can be highly effective and gratifying. Change can happen almost imperceptibly. There are no concrete steps along the way. Look back and see how far you have journeyed from your starting point. Pause and reflect. "Wow, this time last year, we would never have authentically had these conversations about oppression/inequity/othering." "We once talked about the social determinants of health, but now we're asking about the social determinants of health inequity."

From your colleagues' shifting responses in meetings, you'll gain knowledge about how equity work is imbuing the culture. Perhaps the body language in the room oozed discomfort the first time you brought up a difficult matter, and now folx are jumping into that

> IT IS A GRATIFYING FEELING WHEN YOU OBSERVE SOMEONE ELSE ADDRESS THE INEQUITY RED FLAGS THAT CONTRADICT EQUITY GOALS. I GET THE SATISFACTION OF SITTING BACK AND SMILING, SAYING TO MYSELF, "THAT'S EXACTLY WHAT I WAS THINKING."

dialogue on their own. Maybe everyone used to be silent and hesitant, and now they want to talk. These are big changes that took a lot of "take your time and hurry up" energy to propel. Pay attention to the starting point, watch from where you've come, and always ask yourself what progress truly looks like from where you stand. It is iterative—back and forth. Go fast, slow down, but continue to advance.

AFFIRMING ALL OUR STEPS FORWARD AND STEPS BACK

No one can whistle a symphony. It takes a whole orchestra to play it.

—H. E. LUCCOCK

When I accepted my first professional public health position as the newly established AIDS educator, our health department director / health officer was a phenomenal man who became a health officer when he was in his thirties, bringing to the table a worldview shaped by his Peace Corps experiences—his impact continues to influence the actions of the leaders he inspired (like me). I became the second director of the Ingham County Health Department since the tenure of Bruce Bragg, and the two of us built upon his lasting legacy. What we refer to as "the Ingham way" instilled in us the mindset that the *public* in public health was our greatest asset as a department. Our charge was to engage *in* and *with* community in ways that led them to see us as their predominant resource and ally. That was equity leadership before we used the label! It was a leadership value that led to equitable outcomes and continues to do the same even now.

We do this work for today and *in* today, and it continues to follow us into tomorrow. Equity leaders are change makers and culture shifters. As I said in the beginning, this is *legacy* work but is also our work for *right now*. Your leadership will have a profound impact on tomorrow, and it must also act to change our present. I have heard people say that inequity will never change in our lifetime … it is too big. I beg to differ. It has changed. It seems that those who hold the "not in our lifetime" mindset are focused on the outcome—checking that box! But equity leaders who see the critical value in the process recognize that change is happening all around them, despite continuing events that seem to contradict that progress.

One of the aspects of being a senior leader that I've always struggled with is the practice of receiving (or taking credit) for corporate accomplishments. I think, *I didn't actually do that*, while others assure me that I set the tone and priorities, organized the budget investments, and invited the conditions to make it happen. For me, it remains an odd feeling. I have to question what weight I carried to help the team accomplish a particular goal. *Leadering*—I'm moving the change, but this action is so continual that self-congratulation has never felt right, or dare I say "equitable," to me.

However, as equity leaders, we are part of the whole and make sure that our teams have what they need to succeed, including full access to our head, heart, and hands. Our work has a ripple effect. It begins in our hearts and minds, and then it disseminates through our staff and our organization, and ultimately, the community receives the benefit of our efforts. As we intentionally *see*, *say*, and *do* differently, the impact of equity—our collective journey—spreads.

ONGOING, EVER-FLOWING EQUITY

The answer to every adversity lies in courageously
moving forward with faith.

—EDMOND MBIAKA

Not only must we continue to lean into the concept of continuation over conclusion, but we must also resist the urge to jump to conclusions. One strategy for not jumping to conclusions is establishing a keen focus on inequity as well as equity. Margaret Whitehead's definition of health inequity highlights differences in population health status and mortality rates that are systemic, patterned, unjust, and actionable, as opposed to random or otherwise caused by those who become ill. She clarifies that a lack of health equity provides a difference in health outcomes that "are not only unnecessary and avoidable but, in addition, are considered unfair and unjust. Equity in health implies that ideally everyone should have a fair opportunity to attain their full health potential and, more pragmatically, that no one should be disadvantaged from achieving this potential, if it can be avoided."[9]

In this seminal definition, published in 1992, Whitehead does three critical things. She invites values to the table by saying that this practice is unjust. If our national mantra is liberty and justice for all, then those things that are unjust and unfair must be undertaken in our pursuit for equity. The second thing she does in this definition is throw down the action gauntlet! There is absolutely something we can do about this. When others feel that poverty and racism are too big and entrenched for us to fix, our equity acumen can assure us that poverty and racism are socially constructed, made by people, and people have the ability to reverse them. The ongoing, ever-flowing journey of equity requires numerous pit stops to address and shine the light on inequity.

The third thing Whitehead does in her definition is give us hope. Here are the hints to deconstruct the inequities that are getting in the

---

9   Allan Goldberg, "It Matters How We Define Health Care Equity," *Institute of Medicine of the National Academies*, January 18, 2012, https://nam.edu/wp-content/uploads/2015/06/BPH-It-Matters-How-we-define-Health-Equity.pdf.

way of *achieving* equity. The blockades are patterned and systemic. So how do we get to equity? *We seek out inequities that happen over and over, identifying them by the patterns we see. We also look at systems as our starting point for change. We are not flowing with a blindfold covering our eyes. We know where to start and how to continue.*

The celebration of conclusions (i.e., *endings*) is an idea that we are taught. Equity work is iterative and ever changing, and perhaps never ending! The needs are such that none of us can conclude the journey … It took us multiple generations to get to this place, and it will take multiple generations to get us up and *out* of this place. I don't want to hear that change won't happen or that it won't happen in our lifetimes. It is *happening* in our lifetimes, at this very moment. We will see the fruits of our labor, and those rewards will translate into more fuel to move ahead.

WE SEEK OUT INEQUITIES THAT HAPPEN OVER AND OVER, IDENTIFYING THEM BY THE PATTERNS WE SEE. WE ALSO LOOK AT SYSTEMS AS OUR STARTING POINT FOR CHANGE. WE ARE NOT FLOWING WITH A BLINDFOLD COVERING OUR EYES. WE KNOW WHERE TO START AND HOW TO CONTINUE.

I used to say that I do this work so that my children won't have to. Well, I missed that mark. My children are now adults, so my mantra shifted to *I do this work so that my grandchildren won't have to.* Indeed, the work continues. I hold on to the goal of one day sitting on the porch and talking to my grandkids. I'll explain to them what I used to do as a leader and see the confusion on their faces: "What? You had to teach people about race? That's so strange!" Yes, I did, just as people once had to learn that the earth was round …

Our nation and culture are evolving even though some days it feels like we are devolving! This seems to be a slow-paced movement, but we remain fueled with urgency and pace-setting as a strategy. Many researchers seek to create an equity index, but there is still no "official" measurement of equity progress. People naturally wonder, "How do we know when we've arrived as opposed to simply making progress?" I offer that we begin to see shifts around us.

Years ago, in my guest lectures for public health students in various universities, I would ask, "Why are you interested in public health? As master's degree students, what compels you?" I would receive very diverse responses. Some would say, "Oh, I'm interested in environmental health, maternal health, chronic disease, adolescent health, etc." Everyone had a different niche they wanted to affect in various *sectors* of public health. I don't implement this question anymore because over the past five years, when I ask why they are interested in public health, everyone in the classroom says, "I'm interested in health *equity*." Everyone …

That's a qualitative outcome that happened all around me, and I would say that is progress. The mindset of students has moved outside of the silos of specialty public health areas. The students I have spoken to are now focused on foundational, equity-driven work. Transforming public health back to its history of root causes was the goal we articulated in our health equity social justice work at Ingham County during the 1990s, and it appears to now be the goal of a newly empowered workforce! The transformation in the field of public health (and its partner professions) is happening, my friends.

We are the generation that is designing and developing this new norm. If we do it well, those who receive the baton from us will continue to build upon this vital change work. That is continuation over conclusion. I see a *green stop sign* ahead—a sure sign that we should continue on and keep going.

LEARNING LESSONS: CONTINUATION OVER CONCLUSION

- We are socialized, trained, and taught to seek the conclusion—the outcome.
- Baby steps can cover a lot of ground faster than you think.
- We do the work for today, and it follows us into tomorrow.
- Equity is ongoing and ever flowing.

MIRROR MOMENTS: CONTINUATION OVER CONCLUSION

1. What equity principles do you strive for every day that have no designated finish line?
2. Reflect upon a moment when others spoke up about inequity red flags. What factors contributed to this freedom that they felt?
3. When have you been the maverick who said, "No, continuation is what we need in this case and not conclusion?"

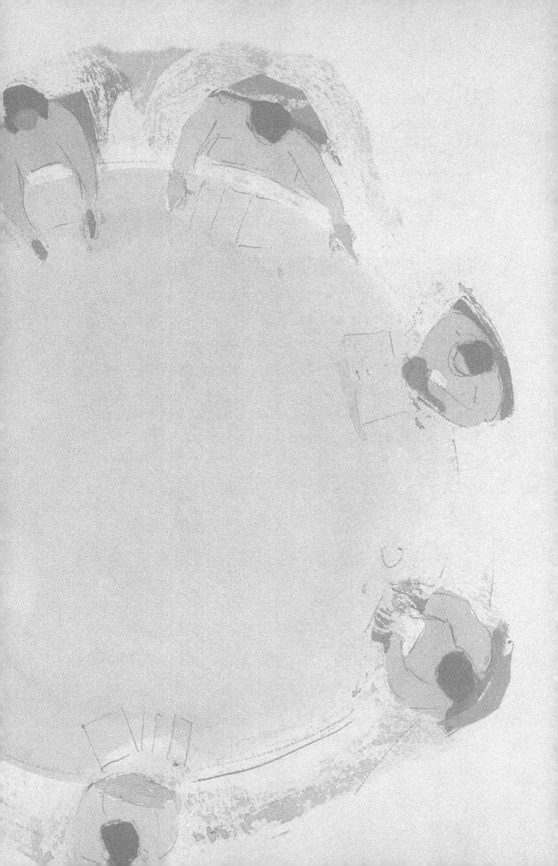

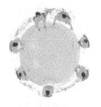

CHAPTER ELEVEN

AKOBEN—A CALL TO ARMS

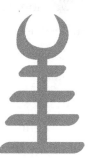

I don't feel no ways tired,
I've come too far from where I started from.
Nobody told me that the road would be easy,
I don't believe He brought me this far to leave me.

—A TRADITIONAL GOSPEL SONG AS PERFORMED BY JAMES CLEVELAND

A s this book comes to a close, I find myself applying introspection and thinking that while books typically end with a conclusion, I have exhorted you to choose continuation over conclusion. So to intentionally unlearn the practice of writing a conclusion, I offer instead a call to arms—we throw down the gauntlet, sound the alarm, and prepare to battle those things that impede the attainment of equity and justice.

The Akoben symbol is an adinkra character from the Asante people of West Africa. The emblem is a war horn, representing vigilance. During the civil rights movement, many songs, poems, and speeches challenged us to hold on, lean in, or keep our eyes on the prize. A call to arms implies an urgency, as opposed to just offering an invitation to join in. A call to arms cries, "Get in there. We need you!"

Our call to arms, as you might expect, is a call to *head, heart, and hands*, but it is also a call to your feet! Hands lift the heavy load of inequity and justice for the sake of the health and well-being for all, but our feet keep us moving. We cannot stand still. We need as much forward momentum as we can leverage. Your hands hold up the work, your head helps you to strategize where you're going, and your heart continually motivates you—driving you on those frustrating days to proclaim, "Nope, I'm not tired. I'm still in it to win it."

It is easy for leaders to be tempted to throw in the towel … Sometimes this manifests as benign neglect as we slip back into old habits. When you consider current systems, reports, models, cultural norms, and all the other elements that determine *how we operate*, most of these function as they always have done. *Business as usual*—sameness, habit, and routine. The beauty of equity transformation is that it is intrinsically about *not* doing things the way they have been done. The budgeting process? Work assignments? Resource distributions? Nothing has changed for decades. So then we apply equity leadership and ask, "What needs to shift?"

As equity leaders, we must continually resist the temptation to devolve into the status quo or an equality response (treating everyone the same). I recall serving on a statewide advisory committee focused on a specific disease condition. During a meeting of partners and organization representatives, the priority of equity and innovation was firmly stated at the opening of the meeting. The agenda then transitioned to brainstorming intervention ideas, and there was no loss of ideas. After listening to the numerous proposals—all enthusiastically received—I presented a simple question to the group: "How do these suggestions represent innovation and equity?"

If we say that we need to be mindful of equity—which everyone seems to be saying—how would our intervention suggestions do that? How do our interventions prioritize *equity* and innovation? If we've been doing things the same way and still have the same inequitable outcomes, it is fair to say that these "solutions" are not working. For far too long, we have clung to what's *easy*, even if *ineffective*. For example, "What can be done within the two-year grant cycle? What can be done without hiring new staff? What can be done without the 'extra effort' of community involvement (because we are the *experts*)?"

How do these suggestions represent innovation and equity? After I offered my question, there was silence and then more silence. As the meeting carried on, others began to refer to the question with comments like "Well, I think it was a good point that Renée made about innovation. What's *different* about how we're approaching this issue … ?" That was the operative question, and the dialogue began to deepen. At times, we have the privilege of preparing the soil; other times, we plant the seed; sometimes we water it; and on occasion, we harvest it. We may not know the role we are playing in the moment, but it is critical that we act, whether the response is in the moment, delayed, or absent.

Accepting the call to arms means never letting yourself off the hook. In your leadership role, you'll likely be presented with several "wonderful" plans and programs. Appreciate their effort, accept their comments, and agitate for equity. Advancing courageous change requires that we stand up and then step forward. Know that you will often experience resistance when you're *adamant* about innovation and questioning the past ... Resistance in others is a call for insistence from yourself (after overcoming the personal hesitance we discussed previously). Your insistence on an equity perspective will often shake people (so expect it). You may silence many rooms. And each time that you do, take pride in the fact that you are enacting what is called for in this moment and this season ...

EXPECTING CHANGE—ADVANCING CHANGE

I've seen too much in life to give up.

—AL SHARPTON

During a partnership between our local health department and one of our local health systems, I bemoaned the challenge of getting my public health colleagues to move beyond the status quo. "If I could just get people to think outside the box," I lamented. My colleague quickly responded, "Think outside the box? I'm just trying to get my clinical colleagues to think outside the bed!" Our context does indeed shape our mental models. In this case, the hospital bed and the bedside manner culture encapsulated priorities and actions. And despite our shared frustration with the resistance to change at the time, we would both admit that change (if even incremental) has happened and is happening.

> EQUITY LEADERSHIP IS NOT ABOUT WHAT WE DO. IT IS ABOUT HOW WE DO WHAT WE DO AND WHY WE DO IT.

Equity leadership is not about what we do. It is about how we do what we do and why we do it. As with the word *equity*, we often see the term *change agent* thrown around. Change agents are both deified and disregarded ...

People look at these problems as far too enormous to overcome. They look for that single person to place on a pedestal who will lead the way. It's an equity issue call, [insert your name!]. Naturally, you won't individually be able to fix racism. You won't individually fix poverty. However, you are not working individually as an equity leader. There is a wave of leaders tackling these issues to the best of their ability in their spheres of influence. Let's return to the undeniable truth: *change does happen.* This is relevant for leaders at every level—town, city, county, state, national, or international—or wherever you are positioned in your organization.

I think often about our civil rights change agents, many of whom were college students. I can imagine that Martin Luther King Jr., Andrew Young, John Louis, Diane Nash, and others sat in hotel rooms thinking, *What are we doing? Are we out of our minds? This is not going to change.* But they also had a deep conviction, knowing that things could and *would* change. Determination and faith pushed them ahead, despite any doubts, fears, and self-interests. They did their part to initiate a revolution of change, knowing that the fruit of their labor would accrue to many. They witnessed change in their lifetimes. We will also see change in our lifetimes as leaders who continue to have hope and believe that the health and well-being of our nation and institutions can evolve. Trust in the inevitability of change—the fruits of your own labor. That inner conviction is the hallmark of a true change agent. It begins with you and your *vision*. Expect and prepare for change.

THE END OF THE BEGINNING

*The greatest glory in living lies not in never
falling, but in rising every time we fall.*

— NELSON MANDELA

I was recently presented with the question "What is our biggest challenge as equity leaders moving forward?"

Five years ago, no one anticipated COVID-19 and the bright spotlight it would shine on the inequities and disparities in our country. Had we been diligently building those equity muscles beforehand, walking the talk and not just talking the talk, we would have better positioned ourselves to do the heavy lifting. Given the disproportionate outcomes, it would seem that our equity work was in a nascent state, but please understand that the beginning stage of our equity work has passed. We can no longer afford to simply see ourselves as novice practitioners in this work.

So I will ask *you*: "What do you think is our biggest challenge as equity leaders moving forward?" This is an agitational question, and the answer comes in the form of another question. "How do we prepare for what's down the road?" Consider the three *wells*:

1. Well-being
2. Well-meaning
3. Well-doing

Well-being, or the state or condition that we are pursuing as related to equity, can be unclear and misdefined. The absence of such clarity threatens solidarity across allies and results in confusion and antagonism across opponents. Therefore, building a shared meaning and goal will also help us to remain accountable to each other and those we serve. Because this is relationship-driven work, we cannot disregard the challenge of those who have good intentions but are risk averse or conflict avoidant (these are **well-meaning** folk). Being well-meaning should also remind us that we are responsible for the intent of our actions as well as the impact of our actions. If we mean well, we should *do* well. A dedication to **well-doing** focuses on the impact of our actions. Are we doing the right things that advance a deep vision of equity? We prepare for the future through *well-being* (a clear goal), *well-meaning* (strong intensions), and *well-doing* (effective impact).

A quote from the book of Galatians says, "Be not weary in well doing." In other words, don't get tired of doing the right thing. Equity leadership can be lonely and taxing, but future generations are depending on us to not throw in the towel. It will be worth it in the end. We're advancing change …

MAKING SPACE FOR QUESTIONS AND QUESTIONING

The master key of knowledge is, indeed, a
persistent and frequent questioning.

—PETER ABELARD

Another unlearning/relearning opportunity: leaders are often socialized to bristle at questions ("How dare they question me!"). But we are learning to invite questions and questioning. As we lead change for equity, we encourage questions and question the questions (are we asking the right things?), and we build space for questioning in our relationships. Asking yourself important questions should become a habit. Similarly, welcoming questions of others helps us then cling to curiosity and disrupt the status quo. How do you also consistently ask questions when no one around you bats an eye at the conditions and contradictions to equity that are so apparent to you? We individually and collectively uncover new ways and opportunities by asking questions.

I was always that child who asked why, a habit that followed me into adulthood. I can accept no for an answer if it is followed by an explanation of why! Little did I know this would be a tremendous skill as a public health professional and a fundamental quality for equity leaders in any field. Keep asking why.

> **WE PREPARE FOR THE FUTURE THROUGH WELL-BEING (A CLEAR GOAL), WELL-MEANING (STRONG INTENSIONS), AND WELL-DOING (EFFECTIVE IMPACT).**

In public health, we apply the quality-improvement method known as "the five whys." This method helps us to uncover root causes—those factors below the surface. The causes of the causes. This straightforward technique allows the answer to the question to position the next *why*. An equity lens pushes us to ask why and get to deeper sources of inequities. For example, the five whys allow us to deepen our approach to difficult questions like *Why are Black maternal deaths twice those of white women? Why are boys of color disproportionately involved in the justice system?* Perhaps even questions at the organizational level like *Why is Black attrition for our company twice that of white attrition? Why is employee engagement with staff of color significantly less than with white staff?*

Our work *is* action … and the right action can come from asking *why*. Keep asking why until you get far enough upstream to understand the foundational cause of any situation. In public health, upstream work has to become mainstream. The social determinants of health—housing, education, employment, healthcare, neighborhoods, etc.—are *midstream*, at best. We have been intervening in these areas for years, without addressing matters of equity and the racism, classism, or gender oppression that have contributed to the inequitable patterns we observe and experience.

Another strategy for going upstream is questioning the very questions that we center and focus on. "Why do people smoke?" is an honorable public health question, but it is an incomplete question. We should also ask questions like *What social conditions and economic policies predispose people to the stress*

> **QUESTIONS LEAD TO DIALOGUE, DIALOGUE IS DOING, DOING IS ACTION, ACTION LEADS TO CHANGE.**

that encourages smoking as a coping strategy? Questions lead to dialogue, dialogue is doing, doing is action, action leads to change. Ask why—confidently and competently, intentionally and vigilantly! We are needed as equity leaders. *You* are needed. This is your call to arms …

LEARNING LESSONS: A CALL TO ARMS

- This is "in our lifetime" work—change is coming.
- Well-being, well-meaning, well-doing—fueled by intent and impact.
- Why not ask why? Ask, and keep asking.

MIRROR MOMENTS: A CALL TO ARMS

1. Where are you needed? Where are you being called upon to be an equity leader?
2. In your current role, how do you make more room at the table for the varied voices and broad beliefs that can help advance equity?

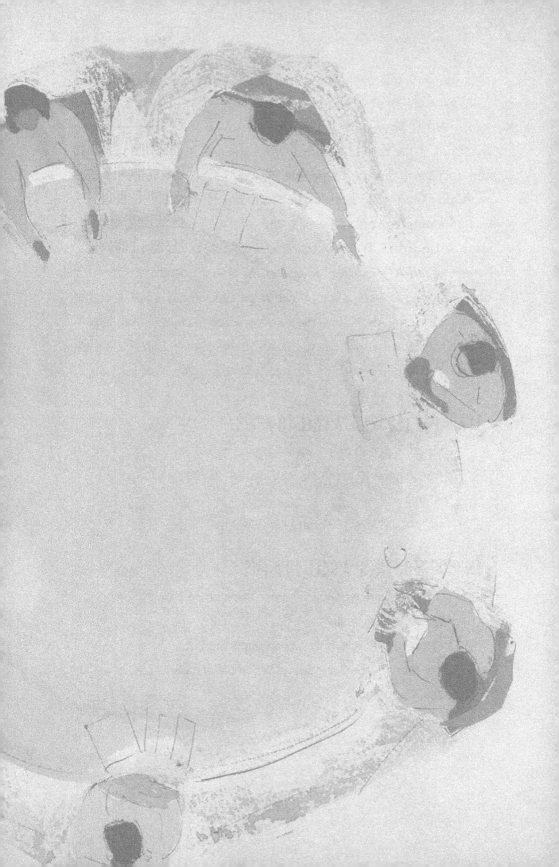

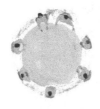

THE INIQUITY OF INEQUITY

iniquity:

gross injustice; lack of justice.

inequity:

lack of equity; injustice; unfairness.

There is no getting around the similarity and iterative nature of the definition of these two words, as well as the fact they are differentiated by only one letter. That distinguishing second *i* in *iniquity* seems to call upon us to peer deeply within—*Am I contributing actively or passively to the very thing I say that I want to help eliminate?* The word *iniquity* triggers our moral compass. Our intentions, or even natural inclinations, are to avoid iniquity. How are we allowing that drive to motivate

AM I CONTRIBUTING ACTIVELY OR PASSIVELY TO THE VERY THING I SAY THAT I WANT TO HELP ELIMINATE?

our actions and priorities as leaders? The *e* in *inequity* links the concepts of inequity and equity. You cannot accomplish equity without uncoupling it from inequity. That requires us to face and disrupt inequity—a task I am fully persuaded we can accomplish.

SO WHAT?—NOW WHAT?

> *The impatient idealist says: "Give me a place to stand and I shall move the earth." But such a place does not exist. We all have to stand on the earth itself and go with her at her pace.*
>
> —CHINUA ACHEBE

So what? Here we are at the final pages of this journey. If you are holding this book, you have privilege. You are likely employed and educated. You may not be a senior leader, but you are a leader nonetheless. You may be a man, you may be a Christian, or you may identify with some other social identity that has been historically valued above others in this country. Peggy McIntosh refers to this as "unearned privilege." Nothing to feel guilty about or ashamed of but also a fundamental call to awareness that can be used to advance change. You have a sphere of influence and impact. In our selah moment, you may not feel that you have been equipped with all the answers you had hoped for, but you can gain comfort in your ability to invite and hold the questions that will advance dialogue and change.

In the interest of dialogue, while it is important to build a shared vocabulary with our partners, don't allow yourself to be distracted by the shiny things—the *latest* word, phrase, or label of the day. When I was a new public health professional battling the discrimination and oppression experienced by those diagnosed with AIDS, we did not call it *inequities* or *social determinants of health*, but that was exactly what we were dealing with (battling, grappling, living through productive outrage!). I fully expect that the future will again bring a shift in the words chosen to describe the phenomenon discussed in this book, but the need for equity-driven room at the table remains.

In the current vernacular is our equity leadership work about antiracism or antioppression? Yes! Both/And! I advocate for the use of the term *antioppression*, recognizing that, especially in the US, racism is the root of most institutional and structural systems that engrain a hierarchy of human value. Our antioppression frame addresses racism explicitly but not exclusively. It also makes room at the table for other forms of oppression—building solidarity across our differences, regardless of the label du jour. The only answer to "Now what?" is keeping our hands on the plow of equity work.

> **IN THE CURRENT VERNACULAR IS OUR EQUITY LEADERSHIP WORK ABOUT ANTIRACISM OR ANTIOPPRESSION? YES! BOTH/AND!**

DO OR DIE (OR DEI!)

> *The essence of global health equity is the idea that something so precious as health might be viewed as a right.*

> —PAUL FARMER

Once upon a time, in a land near and dear, the phrase most commonly used was "diversity and inclusion." Upon further passage of time, the collective construct morphed to "diversity, equity, and inclusion." I often find myself pragmatically wondering why *equity* was the last guest invited to the party, and more illuminating still, why the word was positioned in the middle of the phrase. Why is the acronym DEI and not DIE? I can imagine another conference room meeting where someone says, "Well, we can't say 'DIE'—that would be terrible branding …" I beg to differ! Perhaps seeing the DIE acronym may be just the provocation and agitation that we need to proclaim that there are practices and worldviews that quite candidly need to die and become things of the past.

It won't surprise you that I would prioritize *equity* as the operative construct in this trifecta of DEI/DIE. *EID*, perhaps! Our Muslim friends and partners would tell us that the word *Eid* means celebration. Indeed, aren't we striving for the day when we celebrate the clear presence of equity in the culture of our society? Speech writers would posit that the final point is typically the most important. That puts us back at the DIE acronym. I am not lobbying for an acronym shift, but I am encouraging us again to be intentional in saying what we mean and meaning what we say in order to shift mental models and systems. Remember, we are seeing, saying, and doing differently.

TAKING ON THE MANTLE

Public health is a powerful tool to level that playing field,
to bend the arc of our country away from distrust and
disparities and back towards equity and justice.

—LEANA S. WEN

We're standing on the shoulders of giants: John Lewis, Cesar Chavez, Dolores Huerta, James Chaney, Andrew Goodman, Michael Schwerner, Martin Luther King Jr., Andrew Young, Diane Nash, and so many other courageous leaders who went before us. There is comfort in knowing that we did not begin this work. We were not the ones who laid the foundation, and we may not be the ones who stage the home after it is completely built. Our work is somewhere between those two vital construction events. But a leadership mantle has been left for us by those whose names we know and many, many more whose names we will never know.

Our work is situated during a precarious time that threatens to see a generation with more fear-driven bias and racism than the prior generation. It was previously a truism that the generations of our grandparents and great-grandparents were more biased/racist than subsequent generations. *While current events bring that trajectory into question, they are not our excuses for retreat but rather for active, focused engagement.* How do we take up the mantle? We read, learn, and share dialogue, and we act …

French aviator Antoine de Saint-Exupéry said, "If you want to build a ship, don't drum up people to collect wood and don't assign them tasks and work, but rather teach them to long for the endless immensity of the sea." Health equity is that endless immensity of the sea. It is that vibrant place that sustains and shapes our lives. Your role—rather, your **duty**—as a leader is to cast the vision that inspires and motivates those across the sphere of your influence.

> **WHILE CURRENT EVENTS BRING THAT TRAJECTORY INTO QUESTION, THEY ARE NOT OUR EXCUSES FOR RETREAT BUT RATHER FOR ACTIVE, FOCUSED ENGAGEMENT.**

Saint-Exupéry's words charge us to "do differently!" Don't be obsessed with the outcome ("We have to build a ship!") and resist the temptation to delegate and micromanage ("I need a team to find the wood, cut the wood, collect the wood, distribute the wood, account for the wood, and on and on!"). This work is not transactional. It is *relational.* It is *transformational.* It is an *achievable* longing.

ROOM AT THE TABLE

But when you are invited, go and sit down in the lowest
place, so that when he who invited you comes he may say
to you, "Friend, go up higher." Then you will have glory
in the presence of those who sit at the table with you.

—LUKE 14:7-11

You know me now through my storytelling. I have the privilege of serving on several boards of directors. There is a common practice of board members being seated at a long conference table or some other arrangement of "board seats" while staff are seated along the wall or in some other area of the room. Organizations do this all the time. But when we see differently, we can't unsee what we have seen! And once we see it, we are obligated to do or say something. In one such meeting, I decided it was an EMB ("Excuse me, but …") moment. I shared that the segregation of staff and board was ironic, especially given our agenda item on equity practices within this organization. We were manifesting precisely what we said we were seeking to avoid and change. The response from one of my colleagues was "Well, we have it arranged this way so that the board members can be seen on camera," and they added, "The microphones are placed in just the right position to hear the board members."

As is seen in many cases of systemic oppression, structural barriers are put in place to maintain those norms. The unspoken assumption in those excuses/explanations is that staff do not need to be on camera or heard via microphones. If there is a practice that we've been upholding because it is the way that it has always been done or because the structures require it, that is a clear indicator of an opportunity for disruption and change. If we want to be intentional, we have to disrupt structures that reinforce the status quo.

The response to my comments exuded a bit of impatience and slight irritation in classic "It's not that big of a deal …" flare. But I beg to differ. *If there is literally no room at the table, there is probably no room at the table figuratively. Go through the effort to enlarge the table (bring in more chairs, extend the space by juxtaposing another table, etc.). Shifting the structure is undeniably preferable to excluding voices if we are indeed pursuing equity.*

IF THERE IS LITERALLY NO ROOM AT THE TABLE, THERE IS PROBABLY NO ROOM AT THE TABLE FIGURATIVELY. GO THROUGH THE EFFORT TO ENLARGE THE TABLE (BRING IN MORE CHAIRS, EXTEND THE SPACE BY JUXTAPOSING ANOTHER TABLE, ETC.). SHIFTING THE STRUCTURE IS UNDENIABLY PREFERABLE TO EXCLUDING VOICES IF WE ARE INDEED PURSUING EQUITY.

While I imagine that the room setup will be unchanged during our next meeting, it is important to manage my personal impatience or frustration as we facilitate change. Frustration can easily tempt you to leave the table—or paralyze you as you *remain* at the table. Leaving is the easy choice. Shutting down is the easy choice. Or in a more constructive response, frustration can fuel your productive outrage. It can be the energy that prevents you from becoming wary or weary of doing the right thing.

Equity leaders must be willing to stay and agitate to advance change. *You are supposed to be in the room and at the table.* If not, who will ask the tough questions? Who will push? You have an assignment to fulfill and a contribution to make as we unravel the status quo and foster a new tomorrow—a tomorrow with more than enough room at the table.

SELAH AND CONTINUE ON ...

1. Review all your Mirror Moments. What has shifted in your feelings, thoughts, and opinions?

2. From your current standpoint, what strategies can you use to keep people whole and keep them at the table?

3. Repeat after me: "I want to. I get to. I have to!"

4. Recognize the privilege and responsibility of your role at this moment. Where are you needed? Where are you being called upon to be an equity change agent?

5. Is there room at your table?

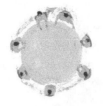

ABOUT THE AUTHOR

Renée Branch Canady, PhD, is a relationship-driven leader who has battled injustice in health throughout her thirty-plus years of public health practice. A recognized national thought leader in the areas of health inequities and disparities, cultural competence, and social justice, Dr. Canady is a sought-after national speaker. She has been influential in broadening health equity/social justice dialogues while serving on national boards, review panels, and advisory groups. Dr. Canady serves as CEO of MPHI, a nationally engaged public health institute in Michigan, and was the Health Officer/Director of the Ingham County Health Department in Lansing, Michigan, where she led the development of the nationally known Health Equity Social Justice program. She continues to serve on the faculty at Michigan State University, where she developed and teaches the public health course on health equity practice.

Dr. Canady is a member of Alpha Kappa Alpha Sorority, Inc., and the Links, Inc., and she is a minister at the Tabernacle of David Church. The mother of three adult sons, all of whom are alumni of Morehouse College, Dr. Canady earned her PhD in medical sociology from Michigan State University, her master's in public administration from Western Michigan University, and a bachelor's in public health nutrition from the University of North Carolina at Chapel Hill.

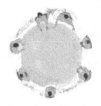

ACKNOWLEDGMENTS

I want to acknowledge the many public health fellows, mentees, and early career colleagues whom I have been honored to encourage and challenge, and who pushed me to put pen to paper. Namely, the Health Equity Awakened fellows and my colleagues at Human Impact Partners who planted the early seeds.

I am thankful to my MPHI family, who were some of my greatest cheerleaders on the journey to completing this book. They celebrated my efforts when I second-guessed myself. My board of directors provided moral and tangible support for this project. I am grateful to them as well.

I am relationship driven because I learned to do *relationship* in a family deeply steeped in love. We love well, fight well, reconcile well, and unconditionally support each other.

I am grateful for my brothers and their amazing wives, their wonderful adult children (my nephews and niece), and the precious great-grandchildren of our family. "HE is the vine; we are the BRANCHES." Much of this book was written by my father's side from his hospital room, then in his rehab center room, and ultimately, in his living room. I remain a "Daddy's girl." I also remain a passionate and committed "boy mom" to three men who push me, encourage me, correct me, lift me, and love me. You are the fuel that drives me to advance equity, and you are the greatest manifestation of God's love for me.

As a mom of boys who also has only brothers, my sister-friends and "sorors," and god-given daughters hold me accountable for my words and actions. We pray together, laugh together, think together, and dream together. Thank you all. I especially acknowledge my friends and colleagues whose skin, race, religion, or perspectives are different from mine and who allowed difference to strengthen and not divide our relationships. You stretch my perspective and embolden me.

I offer a special acknowledgment to my team at Advantage Media Group for being amazing. They taught me so much about expressing myself. As a sociologist, the collaborative nature of this project was an important contributor to its completion. I am especially grateful to Annette Parks and Nate Best. I could not have done this without you!

Printed in the USA
CPSIA information can be obtained
at www.ICGtesting.com
JSHW021629131123
51980JS00003B/36